"Doctor, I feel funny"

How to take the stress out of being in hospital, for patients and visitors

by

Patricia Cameron-Hill & Dr Shayne Yates

Cartoons by George Haddon

Published by Argyle Publications

Copyright © Cameron-Hill & Yates 1999

Editorial by Patricia Cameron-Hill & Shayne Yates

Cover design by George Haddon and Associates

Book design and artwork by David Ely

Copy Editing by Jean Wyldbore, Lucy Malouf and Yasna Blandin de Chalain

Produced through The Talent Bank

Pre Press by The Image Company

Printed and bound in Australia by Griffin Press

ISBN 1 876335 06 8

Available through booksellers and other resellers across Australia.
For further information contact Patricia Cameron-Hill & Shayne Yates
on 03 5472 1976.

Note

This book is sold with the understanding that the content is of a general nature and does not constitute medical, legal, or other professional advice for any specific person or situation.

Readers planning to act on the recommendations made by the authors should first seek professional advice from their doctors, specialists, and other advisors to ensure that such action is appropriate to the reader's circumstances.

Acknowledgements

The book you hold is the work of many hands. We are grateful to all those patients, visitors and health care workers who gave us the benefit of their experience to help with this book.

Our precious thanks to:

Those creative nurses who are prepared to risk trouble to humanise hospitals for patients, visitors and staff. These nurses run punctuality competitions for doctors, let pets visit patients, tell funny stories, massage patients, bring in doughnuts for the night staff, say 'thank you' with chocolate frogs, fish or gold stars, and wear wacky clothes to celebrate special days.

Health care professionals with a special interest in each chapter: for their information and their courage to stand by their point of view.

Francis Macnab for his uplifting sermons, his books and his willingness to contribute to this book his thoughts on faith and fear.

Our many teachers and the authors who have shared their research, experience and ideas on the subject of health and healing. We are especially grateful to the late Dr Norman Cousins for alerting us to the power of the mind-body connection and laughter in healing.

Patch Adams who, by his example, inspired us to finish this book and challenged us to find ways to work harder to serve others. Having experienced for ourselves the benefit and joy of his wisdom, it has given us much pleasure to include some of his wisdom for you, the reader.

George Haddon, our gifted cartoonist, who supported the idea of this book from the start and found the time to make it funny for you and for us.

Taylor Holst, founder of the Australian Humanitarian Foundation, whose unlimited enthusiasm and energy fanned our optimism for making this book available throughout the world!

And finally, Robyn Handbury, for her love, belief in our work and the need for this book. She willingly assumed the role of cheer-leader and organiser, with great tolerance of our writing and working eccentricities!

Patricia Cameron-Hill
Shayne Yates
Castlemaine, Victoria
April 1999

By

Patch Adams, MD

A hospital is a large, very complex, often scary and impersonal institution. It overwhelms most who come into it. You would hope for a sanctuary, a welcoming place...a healing environment...

On the contrary, the rumour is that hospitals are not user-friendly. In illness, needing hospitalisation, the patient is often vulnerable, frightened and anxious. Anything that can relieve these discomforts can make the hospital visit more healing for the patient.

Patricia Cameron-Hill and Shayne Yates have made a fun map for this journey. With their extensive background in human relations and education in the healing arts, they have looked at each part of the hospital stay (and the visitors and staff) and suggested how we can all play a part to improve it. Most of the information is practical and some is there just to make it more fun.

There is something about being sick that makes a person look more closely at the details of their life; as some kind of house cleaning. This is a good book for sick people to read, as it accommodates much of this 'house cleaning' and makes it normal.

On the other hand, it is also a good book for people who are not sick, so that the breadth of all it encompasses will be part of their common knowledge.

So, just as the hotel is expected to have a Gideon's Bible in the bedside table to help guide the traveller in life, so the hospital might put *Doctor, I Feel Funny* in the incoming patient's hand, to help navigate the experience. Thank you Patricia and Shayne for helping to take the stress out of being in hospital.

April 1999

Patch Adams, MD is the founder/director of the Gesundheit Institute, a twenty-seven-year-old project to create a hospital that addresses all the problems of care delivery. The Institute has never charged money, accepted third party reimbursement, or carried malpractice insurance. It is the first hospital to fully integrate all the healing arts and to be wellness- and arts-focused. The hospital is home to staff and patients. It is the first 'silly' hospital in history. In addition, the Institute is now part of its own developing 'eco village'.

Patch Adams is the author of *Gesundheit* (Healing Arts Press), which Universal Pictures has made into the movie 'Patch Adams', starring Robin Williams as Patch himself.

*"Tell you what, you need enormous reserves of good
humour to cope with hospitals these days."*

Patient

Say the word 'hospital' and everyone has a story. These stories are drawn from the treasure trove of human experiences - sad, glad and sometimes funny - that are a part of those wonderful places called hospitals.

Some patients sing the praises of the staff or marvel at what medicine 'can do these days' or give details of their disease and the way it was treated. Others are glad to get out of the hospital and can't wait to get home 'to a bit of peace and quiet and my own bed!'

Visitors have their own stories from their experience of being on middle ground - neither the patient, nor the staff. They see much they should question and some do, but the majority will say, "I didn't like to interfere, it wasn't my place."

Staff have their stories too, though rarely of life and death. More often they talk about who they're working with, where they're working and how busy it is. Stories abound of frantic shifts and not enough staff and what they'd like to do to politicians if it was legal...

Our story is the reason for this book. We love hospitals. We think they are exciting and entertaining and sometimes (often in retrospect) very funny. Working in a hospital, no two days are the same. Each day is filled with the challenge of variety and the element of surprise. The film and television industry knows this of course, and so do the viewers, given the high ratings for hospital drama.

More than the excitement of hospitals, we love hospitals because of the great things achieved in them by dedicated and daring staff. Most of the time they manage to deliver the right treatment, to the right patient, at the right time. No mean feat, considering the number of people and systems that have to be cranked up, with very little notice, 24 hours a day!

Our concern, and the reason for writing this book, is the stress of being in hospital today, whether as a patient, a visitor or a member of staff. Patients don't always know what's going on, visitors sometimes don't know how best to help, and staff are having trouble handling the pressure. Hardly an environment for healing!

In day surgery centres, patients may be exposed to hospital stress for a shorter time, but they can take the stress home with them when they have to manage their own recovery.

The ideas in this book will take the stress out of being in hospital and make the environment more conducive to health and healing. As a patient, you can use these ideas to feel more informed, comfortable, and active in your treatment and recovery. As a visitor you will see the part you can play in the healing process and how to assist the patient in hospital and at home.

The purpose of this book is also to show staff where the opportunities are to reduce stress in hospitals and how to take advantage of them. These opportunities do not require heroic confrontations with the system, but commonsense actions that can be taken at unit or ward level. Actions that will not only benefit the patients and visitors, but will also make working in hospitals more effective and enjoyable.

To make reading this book easier, start by picking a chapter that interests you, then just dip into the rest. Happy reading!

Patricia Cameron-Hill
& Shayne Yates

The impact of hospitalization could be likened to that of being shipwrecked on strange shores: immediate escape is difficult or impossible, the future is unknown but threatening, human contacts are unpredictable but will probably be prone to misunderstandings, the customs and ways of the people yet to be encountered are unknown and likely to be anticipated with apprehension.

Athol Congalton

Contents

Contents

Chapter 1

A highly successful opening

–Your operation

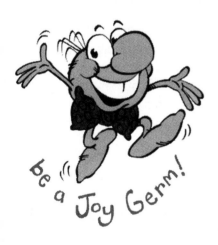

be a Joy Germ!

MOST PEOPLE HAVE attended important openings in their time. But the most important opening you'll ever have as a patient is your own. If you're on the receiving end of the scalpel then you'll agree there are only two kinds of operation - other people's and your own. When other people have surgery they simply have 'an' operation. When you're involved personally it becomes *YOUR* operation - personal and profound.

Keep in mind also that there is no such thing as a minor operation if you're the one being operated on. The doctor may think it's minor, the cleaner may think it's minor, your friends who've had their own operations may think it's minor (compared with theirs) - but it's *your* body and you know differently!

REDUCING PRE-OPERATIVE AND POST-OPERATIVE STRESS

The operation itself is a source of physical stress for the body, especially if you have a general anaesthetic. The process of preparing for the operation, having it, then recovering is also stressful for your mind and body. Being aware of this, there are certain things you can do to reduce the impact of this stress and to promote your own healing. By using the information in this chapter you will know what to expect and how to prepare. This will be a lot more reassuring than listening to people telling you not to worry and to 'just relax'.

Visit the operating theatre

Most hospitals encourage prospective patients to visit the operating theatre/s and the recovery area/s before their operations, because the familiarity will help patients to feel more relaxed. Arrange a time with the staff. They will welcome you and answer any questions you may have.

They don't make 'em like us any more - maybe that's why repairs take a bit longer.

Doctor to patient: "Your condition is so rare, we're not even sure we're pronouncing it right."

RELAX WITH MUSIC

I listened to Mozart before my operation and every
time I heard it I told myself "This is healing music."
Then I played it again straight after the operation
so my mind would associate it with healing.

Patient

While you may expect to be fully asleep and feeling nothing during your surgery, the reality is that your subconscious is still awake and functioning. Our subconscious minds are sponges that absorb all manner of messages which in turn create our attitudes to most things. If the message your subconscious mind is absorbing during surgery is soothing - one that is positive and relaxing - then your body will respond in the same way. (This is the 'mind/body' connection.)

You may like to prepare an audio cassette of your favourite, relaxing music - say 45 minutes each side. Make sure you put your name on the tape, and then give it to the nurse in charge of the operating theatre. Ask that it be played continuously during your operation. The music may be played on a speaker or it is a good idea to bring your own personal cassette with headphones.

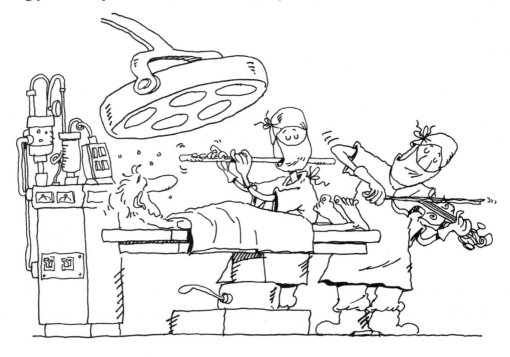

Positive thinking

Talk to your body before surgery. This sounds weird, but it really works. For example, 'We're going to have an operation to help us get well again. We will be relaxed and in good hands. All is well.'

You may even ask your surgeon to speak to you during the operation (even if you're unconscious - because the subconscious mind is always listening). Ask him to speak with hope and encouragement.

GET YOUR BODY IN GOOD SHAPE

Stop smoking as soon as you know you must have an operation. The benefits to your circulation and breathing will be proportional to the length of time you've quit.

It's easy to miss meals and get dehydrated with the preparations and tests required for surgery. So **eat good food and drink plenty of water** before you 'fast'. This will prepare your body for the trauma of surgery and the subsequent healing process.

Once in hospital, if you miss a meal because you're out of the ward, ask for one when you get back.

If you are **having day surgery**, eat well at home the day before.

Keep moving as much as possible before you are prepared for the operating theatre. It's a good time to practise any exercises you'll have to do after the operation.

LOCAL ANAESTHETIC

With local anaesthesia you will be awake during the operation or procedure. This involves making the operation area numb, usually by an injection near the site. You may also have a sedative injection or a tablet to help you relax.

GENERAL ANAESTHETIC

This means you will be unconscious during the operation. You will be given an injection in the ward before you go to the theatre to calm you and relax your muscles. This is called a 'premedication', or 'premed'. (It may also cause a dry mouth and make you drowsy.) Your bedrails may be put up for your safety.

Handy Hint: *It's a good idea to go to the toilet just before your premed, because you'll have to remain in bed after the injection.*

WHAT TO EXPECT BEFORE YOUR OPERATION

Tests may be done in the hospital or before you are admitted. They may include blood tests, X-rays and urine tests.

A visit from your anaesthetist

This person is the doctor who will give you the anaesthetic. Expect a visit from an anaesthetist before your operation to assess your physical state. You may be asked about smoking, alcohol use, medications, past illnesses, allergies, etc. Your responses, combined with your medical record, will help the anaesthetist to build up a picture of your potential response to anaesthesia.

This is the time to mention your relaxation music and also any minor thing you think just may be of importance - like the fact that you're one of those rare people to whom morphine is a stimulant. (It's always preferable if someone is asleep during the operation - and most parties would vote on it being the patient!)

A visit from your surgeon; your consent

Your surgeon may visit personally (especially if you're in a private hospital), or have a junior colleague do so. A **signed consent form** for your operation will be requested from you so that the doctors can go ahead with the procedure. This may happen in the doctor's surgery or in the hospital.

It is a legal requirement that the person who is operating or performing a procedure on you explain what is going to be done and why; what to expect before, during and after the procedure or operation. Risks and possible complications should be included.

If you are unsure, don't sign the form - ask for more information.

Physiotherapist

Depending on the nature of your surgery, a physiotherapist may visit to give you pre-operative exercises and show you what to do after your operation. If a physiotherapist is not available, you can always hire one privately.

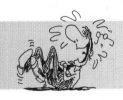

Did you know that hospital gowns were designed by an architect?
That's why they all have a southern exposure.

A nurse may -

- **Shave** your operation site or ask you to do it.
- **Request that you shower** with special soap.
- **'Fast' you** by removing your water jug, putting a 'Nil orally' or 'Nil by mouth' sign on your bed, and asking you not to eat or drink after this time.

  Handy Hint: *Have a big drink before they take your water jug.*

- **Ask you to wear a gown and cap.** The gown ties at the back. For privacy and comfort, wear two gowns, the first one tied up the back, the second up the front.
- Give you **an enema or rectal suppository** to empty and cleanse your lower bowel.

  Handy Hint: *Ask if you can wear disposable or cotton briefs to the operating theatre. They can be removed there.*

- **Ask you to remove:** nail polish, jewellery, lipstick, prostheses (artificial body parts) and dentures.

  Handy Hint: *If you feel strongly about leaving your teeth in, ask if they can be left in place until you reach the operating theatre. Same goes for a special ring - ask the staff to tape over it rather than remove it.*

Before you leave for the operating theatre the nurses will make a check of your name against your ID wrist band, remove or tape jewellery, etc. You may have to move on to a special trolley to go to the operating theatre.

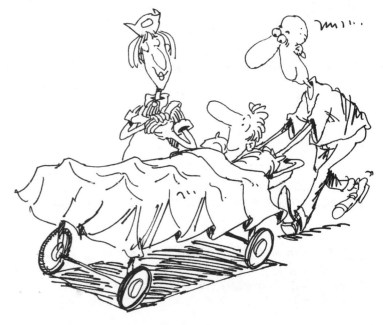

In the operating theatre...

You will be 'checked in' by the staff. They will ask your name, check your ID band, look at your file. We suggest you also mention the name of your operation and the position, for example 'right eye', 'left knee', etc.

Handy Hint: *Trust these people to take good care of you. They know their jobs and are brilliant at them.*

Prepare for a long and pleasant sleep ZZZZZZZzzzzzzzzzzz

AFTER YOUR OPERATION

> *When I woke up, I thought I was still waiting for my operation. It was a great relief to know it was over.*
>
> Patient

You are most likely to wake up in a recovery ward or bay. It is not quite the same as waking up after a night's sleep. Your throat may feel irritated and your mouth dry. You may be a little confused and feel sick. You may have an oxygen mask over your nose, a drainage tube from your wound, a tube (or 'urethral catheter') into your bladder, and/or tubes in your veins ('intravenous therapy').

BACK IN THE WARD

The first time you pass urine is a sign that your bladder is functioning, so use a bedpan or let the staff know you are going to the toilet.

You may not be able to drink and eat by mouth initially, so mouth washes or ice chips to suck are comforting alternatives.

You may have some pain at this time. Pain relief is usually given regularly to start with, then as often as you need it. Keep in mind that this is 'getting well pain', as opposed to 'being ill' pain. **But any pain if unrelieved will cause stress and slow your recovery. So ask for pain relief if you need it,** especially before you go to sleep.

After my operation, I asked the doctor if my scar would show. He said that would be entirely up to me.

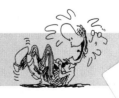

21

Some time later...

Tiredness, 'the blues', and an inability to concentrate for long periods are all common after major surgery. **You must give yourself permission to take time to be well again.**

Use your convalescence as a chance to catch up on reading, making phone calls, watching videos (new releases or old favourites) and contemplating your life.

So many things we take for granted - being able to speak, eat and move. I couldn't do any of those, and I just had to accept it and concentrate on getting them back.

Patient recovering from a car accident

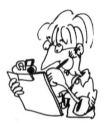

NOTES FOR STAFF

Increasingly, research studies show an important relationship between how a patient feels mentally, and their response to surgery. Fear and panic weaken the immune system and compromise the recovery process. Giving information reduces this fear, reduces stress and helps the patient to feel reassured, relaxed and ready for surgery. Remember, nothing is 'routine' if you're the patient!

Did you hear about the doctor who went into the kidnapping business?
He failed - no one could read the ransom notes!

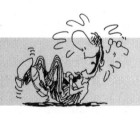

KEEP MOVING!

Along with rest and nutrition, exercise is a key aspect of recovery. When you are in the same position for any length of time your circulation can become sluggish and your breathing shallow. Exercise improves your intake of oxygen and circulation of the blood - both vital for healing and recovery. Exercise can also improve the quality of your sleep. A little exercise will also stimulate your appetite, keep you 'regular', and improve your bladder control.

Your mental state can also benefit from physical exercise; it can lift your mood and give you more energy. No doubt this has something to do with your increased oxygen intake but it is also likely that doing something for yourself to assist your own healing contributes greatly to these benefits!

How much exercise do you need?

Every patient needs some movement on a regular basis. Some exercises you can do on your own, but others will need the assistance from physiotherapists or nurses - especially if you have had major surgery.

Movement is also important for the patient who is unconscious or unable to move, in which case their limbs are moved for them. These 'passive exercises' are essential to improve circulation and prevent muscle contraction.

Breathing - five deep breaths each waking hour!

Deep breathing will ensure a good intake of oxygen and help to prevent a chest infection following surgery.

If possible, sit up with your back supported (or lie comfortably). Rest your hands on your abdomen above your navel and relax your shoulders. Breathe in slowly and deeply through your nose (or mouth if easier), letting your abdomen expand like a balloon. (You'll feel your hands being pushed away if you're doing this properly).

Hold your deep breath for about three seconds, then relax and exhale.

Do this five times, then have a short rest. It will benefit you to repeat the five deep breaths and rest again. (If you take more than five deep breaths in a row you may feel dizzy.)

Handy Hint: *Try to avoid raising and lowering your shoulders during the exercise. When this happens, it means that the air is not getting to the bases of your lungs where most of the blood circulates and oxygen is exchanged.*

'Huffing'

The 'huff' is a similar action to fogging up spectacles! Huffing helps to move any secretions in the outer airways of the lungs up to the central airways, so it can be coughed up. Do two huffs after the deep breathing (above) is completed, then have another rest. Then do one strong cough to clear secretions. One strong cough is better than several small ones. If you can't cough, huffing is better than nothing. Do this every hour if necessary.

Handy Hint: *If this part of the exercise is painful, brace your chest by wrapping your arms around yourself before you cough. If you have a wound, you can place a pillow or folded towel over the incision (for support) with your hands while you huff and cough.*

Exercises to improve circulation and muscle function in the legs

Caution: Check with a physiotherapist or nurse before doing these, especially if you've had surgery:

Ankle alphabet - do anytime and at least every hour
Try drawing the letters of the alphabet - from A to Z - with your big toe and foot. You can do this exercise sitting on a chair (this is best) or in bed. At least do the letter 'I' by pulling your feet back toward you, then pointing them down away from you in a pumping action.

Knee flexion/extension - three times a day
Sitting or lying, cross your legs at the ankles. Then push the lower leg up against the upper leg. At the same time, push the upper leg down hard so the lower leg has to work. Do 10 of these for each leg.

Gentle stretches - three times a day

Loop a towel under your foot and pull gently. Stretch to strain, not pain. Hold for 15 seconds, relax. Do five stretches for each leg.

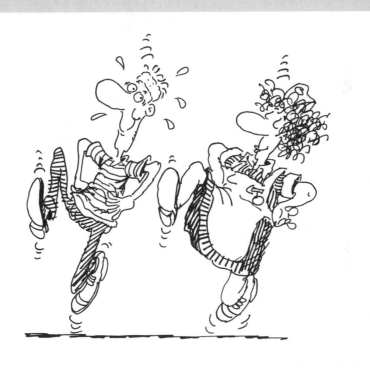

Leg raising - three times a day

Keeping your thigh muscles tight and your leg locked straight, raise and lower each leg off the bed, in turn. Do five raises for each leg.

More Handy Hints

- **Start exercising before your hospital admission.** Check with your doctor or a physiotherapist on what exercises would be most helpful. Something simple and effective is walking. Walk for half an hour, five days out of seven, for at least a month before admission.
- **Walk in hospital** whenever possible if your condition permits. Even if it is just a few steps from the bed to a chair. Ask a nurse or visitor to

assist you to walk the length of the corridor twice a day. To prevent dizziness, sit for a while before you stand after lying in bed. Don't let people rush you!

- **Sit out of bed** as often as possible, but not so long that you feel tired.
- **Get pain relief before a physiotherapy session.** A rest period is also helpful.
- **Be patient and pace yourself.** Healing takes longer than most people think. If you do overdo the exercise it may work against your progress. You need to balance your need for movement with your need for rest.
- **Remember to use a good belly laugh for an internal workout!**

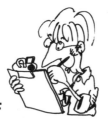

NOTES FOR STAFF

You already know how beneficial exercise is to reduce stress and improve your health. But you may not be aware of the value of just half an hour of brisk walking a day. A major survey showed that this alone can reduce your chance of premature death by 65%!

Exercise can also re-energise you. 15 minutes of brisk walking will give you an energy surge for the next 90 minutes. (This could bring new meaning to a tea break - grab a banana and go for a walk!) We recall a hospital where night nurses were encouraged to take a break during their shift - in the hospital's heated swimming pool! They returned to work feeling less stressed and more alert.

To minimise the chance of back injuries, some hospitals and nursing homes ensure that nurses do exercises, especially stretching, before each shift.

We applaud these hospitals and those that have a gymnasium for staff.

Chapter 2

Going into hospital

– Getting ready

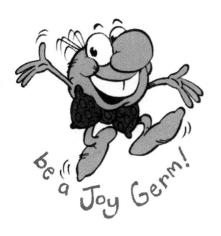

be a Joy Germ!

Be prepared

Before you go into hospital

What to ask the hospital

Before you leave home

What to take with you

Arriving at the hospital

Arriving on the ward

An unexpected or emergency admission

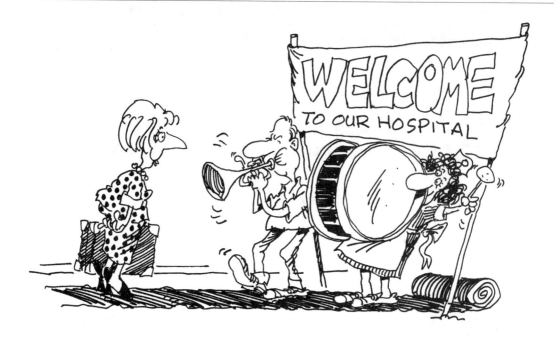

ONE WAY TO take the stress out of going into hospital is to *be prepared*.

- If you are what is called an 'elective' or arranged admission, you'll usually have plenty of time to do this.
- If, on the other hand, you are with someone who has been admitted on an 'emergency' basis, turn to the end of this chapter.
- If you are having day surgery, then we have a special section for you in 'Drive Thru Surgery'.

Which hospital - public or private?

Whether you have private health insurance, and your level of cover, will influence your decision to go to a private or public hospital. Your medical condition also plays a part. If your condition is serious - for example, a heart attack or accident - you are more likely to go to a public hospital. Complex treatments are also a feature of public hospitals which have a range of emergency back-up services and 24 hour cover by doctors. Larger private hospitals, however, have seen the need for these services too and many of them now offer some of the specialised treatments and medical back-up of public hospitals.

If you're having 'elective' surgery (non-urgent) then private hospitals are unlikely to have a waiting list. This means the treatment is faster and you can decide ahead of time when you'll have the surgery or procedure.

If you are put on a waiting list in a public hospital for elective surgery, ask what the expected waiting time is, and if it seems too long, ask whether the waiting list is organised for one particular doctor or for a group of doctors in the hospital - another doctor or another hospital may have a shorter waiting list. Shop around.*

You are also more likely (but not guaranteed) to get a single or private room in a private hospital.

Another factor in hospital selection has to do with what is known as the 'visiting rights' of your doctor - whether or not s/he can use a hospital's facilities.

BEFORE YOU GO INTO HOSPITAL

With shorter hospital stays, hospitals tend to do a lot more patient preparation ('pre-admission procedures') before you're actually admitted. This may involve blood tests, X-rays, a visit to/from your anaesthetist, getting a letter from your doctor, the completion of admission or consent forms, etc. These tasks save time once you're admitted (especially for day surgery), so make sure you do them all and that the results and forms reach the hospital ahead of you or with you.

Visit the hospital

Ninety per cent of the things we worry about never actually happen. And most of these worries usually exist because of lack of information. If you are going into hospital, think about having a look around beforehand. The public relations department should be able to arrange a tour for you. If you do this, you're less likely to feel anxious about or intimidated by the alien surroundings, you'll feel more relaxed, and the staff will be expecting you.

Get information

Most hospitals have 'Information Guides' and some have special instructions for tests and surgery. It's a good idea to have this sent to your home before you go in, or make sure you get it on admission. In larger hospitals there are 'Customer Service' staff or departments who will be keen to help you plan for your hospital visit or stay.

* Choice Magazine, Mar 1996.

WHAT TO ASK THE HOSPITAL

Find out ahead of time about the types of accommodation available - for example, whether you have to share a room, are there bathroom and toilet facilities 'en suite' or are they down the hall, if there is a shared or individual television available, etc.

Whether you are in a public or private hospital, there are single rooms available. In public hospitals they are usually allocated to the sickest patients, but in private hospitals, to the most persistent! However, there are certain advantages in both shared and private rooms.

The advantages of a **private room** are: •Privacy •Quiet •More space.
The advantages of a **shared room** are: •The company •A room mate can be
a life saver in an emergency!

*Patients who are new to hospitals can't realise
how time drags in a room on your own.*

Patient

BEFORE YOU LEAVE HOME

There will always be disruption of family and household routines, no matter who goes into hospital. However, if you are the person who looks after most of the domestic matters, then these ideas may be useful:

- Organise the family and delegate chores. Spell out exactly *what* has to be done, *when,* and *who's* going to do it. You don't want to come home to even more work!
- Order flowers for yourself if you don't expect any!
- Beforehand, eat lots of *good* food, drink plenty of water, and watch some funny videos or movies to help you relax. Get a good night's sleep too!
- Organise redirection of mail and other deliveries if appropriate.
- Don't feel guilty about going into hospital.

WHAT TO TAKE WITH YOU

It may surprise you to learn that it is often the little things that are missing that cause you the most irritation. For example, nurses are very reluctant to hand over their pen to a patient because they suspect they will never see it again! So go through our checklists to make sure that you pack the little things that are important to you.

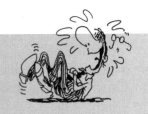

Q. Do you know how long people should stay in a hospital bed?

A. The same as short people.

Remember:

- Soap, toothbrush, toothpaste, shaving kits, razor and tissues.
- Pen/s and notepaper, notelets, postcards, stamps, etc.
- Pyjamas or nightdresses, dressing gown or 'housecoat', slippers.
- Aides you use at home to read, eat, hear, walk, wash, dress, etc.
- Your sense of humour.
- Depending on your condition, you may need lighter or larger clothes to leave the hospital in, than those you were wearing on admission. So organise a set of 'Going Home' clothing, which can be brought to the hospital just before you are discharged.

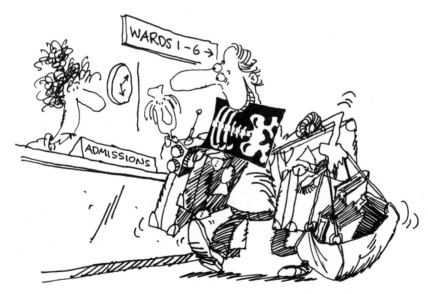

Also take:

- Health fund, MediCare, and any other compensation claim cards.
- Pharmaceutical Benefits Scheme entitlement card.
- Pensioner entitlement card.
- Letter from your doctor.

- Current X-rays.
- Your current medications, including contraceptives, HRT and vitamins.
- Other toiletries: talc, facewasher, brush/comb, cosmetics, mirror, hairdryer.
- Torch.
- Clock or watch.
- Money - some in change, mostly for the phone, drink machine and lolly trolley!

Helpful extras:

- Soap/moisture impregnated towelettes (good to use after bedpans and before meals!)
- Mouthwash.
- Underpants or knickers.
- A medical sheepskin (See Chapter 10).
- Favourite pillow (with coloured pillowslip and name tag).
- Sleeping mask and ear plugs (from the chemist).
- Blue-Tac (or similar) or double sided/removable tape (for putting cards and notes on wall or locker sides - saves room on the top of the locker!)

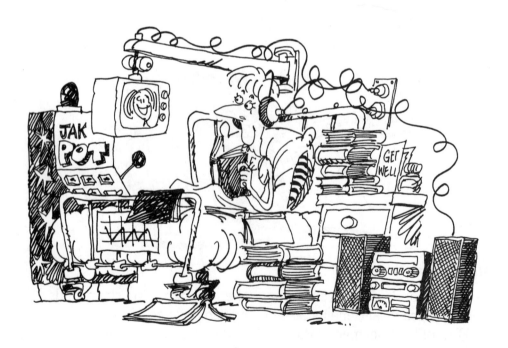

Take some entertainment

Hospitals can switch from being joyful, to boring or miserable, in the space of a few hours. Your energy levels can also vary throughout the day. For example, sometimes reading will be easy, at other times a chore. So take a range of entertainment so that you will have something to distract you no matter how you feel.

- Personal cassette or radiocassette, with earphones and spare batteries.
- Books on tape (from your community library).
- Tapes of favourite music.
- Books - light, happy stories.
- Magazines with lots of pictures.
- Comics.
- Photos of partner, family, pet, favourite place.
- Favourite toy or security blanket (even if you are a 'grown-up'!)
- Personal games and distractions, like playing cards, crosswords, mini jigsaw puzzles, etc.

Don't take:

- Too many clothes (hospitals have limited storage).
- More than about $50 in cash.
- Jewellery that may be lost or stolen (this is your responsibility).
- Electrical appliances such as portable televisions.
- Work to do that's not relaxing!

ARRIVING AT THE HOSPITAL

It is useful if you find out ahead of time where you have to report. It's usually the Admissions or Reception area.

No matter what time you were told to be there, you will be either early or late! So expect delays and be prepared. Find out the approximate waiting time before you're admitted and either settle down with a good book or leave and come back later.

It is likely you will be admitted by the staff in Admissions and your details will be entered in the computer. You'll be given a hospital number or file number, and a wrist band, for identification purposes.

* If you want that private room, now is the time to ask (or phone the day before).

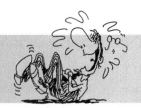

Hope your hospital stay is like the gown they give you -
short and with the end in sight.

ARRIVING ON THE WARD

Expect...

- to be asked to change into your night clothes or hospital gown, even though you feel quite well and it is the middle of the day!
- that a record may be made of clothes and items you've brought with you.
- that your 'observations' will be taken including weight, urine testing, temperature and blood pressure.
- that nurses may take a 'nursing history' to get to know you - tell them about any allergies, reactions to certain medications, previous illnesses or pregnancy.

Make sure you...

- know your way around and can find toilets, phone and exits.
- know how to operate your call bell and bed and that they both work.
- introduce yourself to the other patients near your 'spot'.

Some time later...

In a public hospital, a doctor will arrive to 'admit' you formally. S/he will take your 'history', examine you, write notes and issue instructions to the attending staff. Tell the doctor what you told the nurses about allergies, etc. This is a good time to ask the doctor any questions that you may have about your admission or procedure.

In a private hospital it is likely that this will vary and you may not see your doctor on admission. Ask the unit staff, as they will know your doctor's routine. That way you won't be left wondering if they're coming in or not. It's a good idea not to go roaming about before the doctor 'admits' you - unless it will be several hours!

So settle in, spread out your comforts from home, create your 'healing bedside',
lie back and relax - knowing that you are in good hands.

I'm not looking forward to going into hospital. The moment you
walk through those doors you face your own mortality.

Patient

AN UNEXPECTED OR EMERGENCY ADMISSION

Get involved. Be visible. Take control and ask questions. Don't be intimidated by the staff and what's going on.

Wife of accident victim

An emergency admission can happen at any time, and nothing can prepare you for the shock. It is an emotionally-charged situation, because people are distressed and concerned. If you're the patient, your main worry will be getting something done. If you're with the patient, you may be critical of what is being done, and it's hard to accept that your loved one is only one of many patients being treated.

But remember that the staff are health professionals, who will have quickly assessed the immediate danger to the patient, and be acting appropriately.

You must expect that the police may have to interview you if you've been involved in an accident. They will want your name, address and details of the accident. You have a right to have a solicitor present before answering any questions.

You may also have to wait for attention. Try to find out the approximate waiting time, so you can adjust your expectations and advise family members, and make sure you are not forgotten.

I was left on a trolley in Accident and Emergency for five hours before I worked out what to do about it. I started crying - and I was in the ward in 20 minutes.

Patient

Handy hints:

- Accept your negative feelings and give yourself time to work through them.
- Remember to notify your partner, people who may be expecting you, the rest of the family, as appropriate, or arrange to have them contacted by hospital staff or police.
- Try not to look frightened in front of the patient!
- Maintain your home routines as much as possible, because it helps you to know that some things are in order.
- Let your family and friends know *how* they can help. Not necessarily by visiting but perhaps in other ways, like helping with transport and chores.
- Consider putting 'health bulletins' or 'progress reports' on your answering machine, so people can find out the latest news about you without having to speak with you.

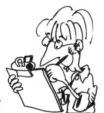

NOTES FOR STAFF

When you work in Accident and Emergency, there is little you can do about waiting time. You can, however, reassure people by letting them know they haven't been forgotten.

Did they really mean that?
From Doctors' dictating machines:

"We have been sitting on this patient for a long time because of his multiple problems."

"By the time she was admitted to hospital, her rapid heart had stopped and she was feeling much better."

"Patient stated that if she would lie down, within two or three minutes something would come across her abdomen and knock her up."

Internet

Chapter 3

"This is not a hotel"

– Hospital life

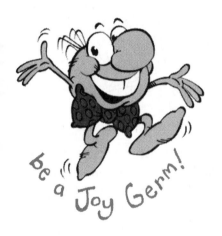

be a Joy Germ!

'Difficult' and 'good' patients

Hours of business

Routines

Who's who

Doctors

Nurses

'Allied Health' staff

Support staff

Volunteers

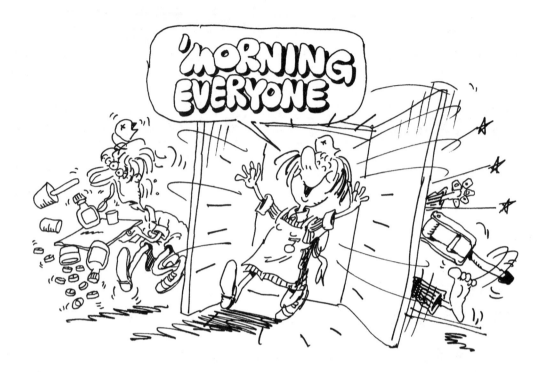

"WHAT DO THEY think this is - a hotel?" This is an expression sometimes used between hospital staff when a patient makes what the staff think is an unreasonable request. This could include asking for a private room (or "One with a view!"), different food (and a cup of tea for the visitor), a vase for flowers, a glass of wine or a telephone. When patients make these requests, they think they are being quite reasonable, especially if they are paying around $500 a day in a private hospital.

In a public hospital, however, although the type of request may differ, it is still likely that some requests will be considered unreasonable. For example, using the ideas and suggestions in this book - many of them fair and achievable - may be considered by *some* staff as unrealistic in a busy hospital.

Whether a public or private hospital, rarely do patients and staff have the same idea of what is going on, nor what each other should be doing. The misunderstandings that result can cause conflict and stress for both patients and staff.

The only good thing about being sick in a hospital is that it gives your credit cards a chance to rest.

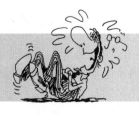

For many people, going into hospital is like going to a foreign country. The words that hospital people use are not familiar. The people dress differently, and there are rules and regulations for everything! The quicker you get to know the language and the way things are done in hospital, the quicker you'll adjust and be able to get what you want. **This book is your 'guide' to that foreign land.**

The first thing to understand about hospitals is that they are organised to suit the people who spend most time there. That is, the staff. You probably thought we were going to say 'the patients'. No! Patients come and go, but the staff spend the most time in hospital. After all, they are always there to look after you.

This is not to say that staff don't *care* about patients. They certainly do, but they must also get their work done. Have you ever wondered why so many patients are woken early in the morning? So the night staff can finish their work and go home.

Your particular needs and wants are vitally important to you, but occasionally in hospital you may hear the expression, "You're not the only one." And you're not! As a patient, you are competing with other patients for the time and attention of the staff. The good news is that the more you understand hospital life from the point of view of the staff, the easier it will be for you to get the attention you need.

'DIFFICULT' PATIENTS AND 'GOOD' PATIENTS

Even though patients may try very hard to 'do the right thing', they may still fall short of what the staff expect of them and so run the risk of being considered 'difficult'. 'Difficult' behaviours include ingratitude, rudeness, manipulation and aggression. But you can also earn this title if you try to take control of your situation by being an 'assertive consumer' - asking questions, challenging treatment, making demands and generally breaking 'The Rules'. (Be consoled - *studies show that 'difficult' patients have a higher survival rate than 'good' patients because they are more likely to have their needs met.*)

In contrast, 'good' patients are those who are really no trouble to look after. They fit into the hospital routine, abide by the rules and ask few questions. They do not sit on their buzzer, and they are grateful for all that is done for them. We have seen many self-confident and assertive people become passive and compliant patients, so that they will be perceived by the staff as no trouble to care for.

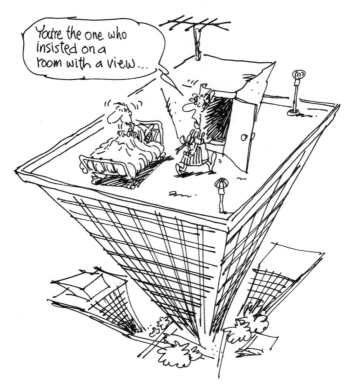

HOURS OF BUSINESS

Hospitals run 24 hours a day, seven days a week. But like any business, some things are easier to get done at certain times. For most departments and services, the hospital works on 'office hours'. If you ask for something between 8 am and not much later than 3 pm, Monday to Friday, you'll have a better chance of your request being met.

'After hours' requests can be met, but it's much more difficult for the staff to help you. At these times hospitals are mainly run by nurses, especially the nursing supervisor. So ask to see this person if you are having difficulty in getting what you want.

I wanted to be liked by the nurses. But the problem caused by being pleasant to the staff all the time was that they underestimated the seriousness of my condition.

Patient

ROUTINES

When there is a lot of work to do, and not much time to do it, the most effective way to get things done is to have set routines. When you go into hospital you will be expected to co-operate with these routines *immediately*. This is typical of most hospitals:

6-7am	Time to wake up, take pills, observations are done, etc.
8am	Breakfast (unless you're fasting!)
8.30am-12 noon	Peak activity time - showers, washes (called 'sponges'), doctors' rounds, treatments, observations done, etc.
9.30am	Morning tea.
12 noon	Lunch.
1-4pm	Some treatments, tests, visitors, afternoon tea. Nurses report to each other at shift changeover (try not to interrupt this!) Patients' rest period (in some hospitals).
4.30-6pm	Evening meal.
6-9pm	Treatments, visitors and supper.
9-10pm	Prepare for sleep, night nurses and low activity (unless your bed is near the nurses' station or corridor!)

WHO'S WHO

There are always lots of different staff in a hospital. Basically they can be divided into two groups. *Health care professionals* (doctors, nurses and 'allied health' staff) and the *support staff* (cleaning, catering, clerical, pastoral care, porters and engineering staff).

Don't be surprised if you don't get the doctor you want.

Public patient

Staff are identified by the cut and colour of their uniforms and this varies from hospital to hospital. If you don't know what job a person in a certain colour does, ask them: "May I know what your job is?" When you have this information you can ask the right person for what you want. If you remember the names of staff as well, it makes them feel important and they will be more helpful to you.

DOCTORS

Doctors have the highest status in a hospital and nurses run a close second.

In a large public hospital you'll have a doctor in charge of you ('consultant' or 'specialist'), and often a 'registrar' (trainee specialist) and an 'intern' or 'resident' (junior doctor), who report to the consultant. You usually don't have any choice about which doctor looks after you in a public hospital, unless you are a private patient. But you can always ask for a second opinion.

In a small public hospital, you may have just the one doctor looking after you. If you are admitted to a private hospital, then you will have the choice of your own doctor. You may not see your doctor very often, so if you do want to see him or her, the best way is to work through the nurses. Whether you are a public or private patient you always have the right to ask for a second opinion.

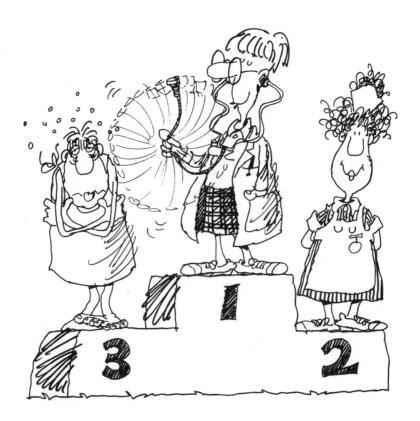

LET'S HEAR IT FOR THE NURSES

The person who can give you the most help in hospital and bend the rules for you is the nurse. Nurses are divided into three shifts in each 24 hours (morning, evening and night), seven days a week. They are assigned specific patients at the beginning of each shift.

It is most likely that you will be looked after by a number of different nurses during your stay. And they may not be the same ones from day to day. So it is very important that you find out who is 'your' nurse for each shift. With so many nurses around it is easy to get confused, especially if you are on medication, so write down their names.

Sometimes you will be looked after by a *relief nurse*. These nurses come from other parts of the hospital or outside agencies, and fill in when needed. Often when a question is asked of a relief nurse, they will reply: "I don't know, I'm just relieving." So be warned, and ask to see someone who *does* know.

I used to wait until my favourite nurse was on duty to ask for things. She was a happy person and smiled a lot.

Patient

'ALLIED HEALTH' STAFF

Ever wondered what 'allied health' really means? This field includes pharmacists, physiotherapists, speech pathologists, radiographers, social workers, podiatrists (who care for feet), dietitians, occupational therapists, counsellors and many more. These people tend to work office hours with a minimal service cover at other times. The usual routine is that your doctor will request that they see you.

It is quite possible that you will not know that the request has been made, until someone arrives at your bed to see you.

If you feel you would like to see one of the 'allied health' staff and your doctor hasn't arranged it, make a request through the nurses.

SUPPORT STAFF

These are the people you'll see most often as they go about their tasks. The cleaners, porters, kitchen and clerical staff. They provide and care for the 'engine room' of the hospital. Without them it would surely grind to a screaming halt. They are usually very helpful and willing to assist, and can add to the success of your hospital stay.

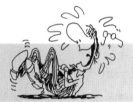

Any place that serves breakfast in bed can't be all bad!

VOLUNTEERS

These people are the *soul* of the hospital. They run the hospital shop, escort patients, arrange flowers, read to patients (or staff!), distribute mail, write and post letters, do shopping, run fêtes, raise money and boost the morale of staff and patients. Ask for them if you need help or a cheering up.

Mother occasionally brought me an egg which was then boiled in the steriliser. Pillows were turned over if an accident should occur and linen was changed once a week! All that has changed these days.

Older patient

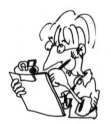

NOTES FOR STAFF

Hospital life is confusing at times for patients and visitors, and also for new staff. We've seen a variety of fun and very creative ways to make our hospitals less stressful for everyone.

Tauranga Hospital in New Zealand has a 'Doorman' to greet and direct patients and visitors. He greets them with a smile, gives information and reassures them.

Here are some more ideas:

- survival kits for new staff and patients; maps; leaflets.
- badges: for new nurse graduates: 'Running In - Please Pass'.
- colourful large print name badges for staff.
- photos of staff on noticeboards - 'Who's Who'.
- 'Welcome' cards.

Fun Slogans (for your specialty)

Coronary Care	*The Beat Goes On*
Orthopaedics	*Smash Repairs, Free Quote*
Maternity	*Keeping Abreast of the Times*
Haemodialysis	*We can Take the Strain*
Gastroscopy	*Light at the End of the Tunnel*
Pastoral Care	*Soul Patrol*
Oncology	*Cytological Support*
Ophthalmology	*We'll Keep a Good Eye on You*
Bone Marrow Transplant	*A Marrowing Experience*
Operating Theatre	*A Cut Above the Rest*
Audiology	*Ear Today, Gone Tomorrow*
Rheumatology	*The Best Joint in Town*

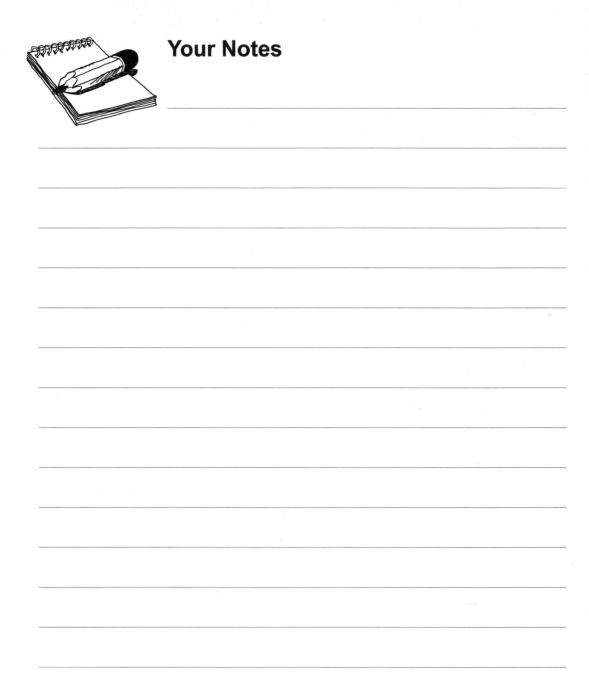

Your Notes

"Oh no! Not more visitors!"

– Managing visitors

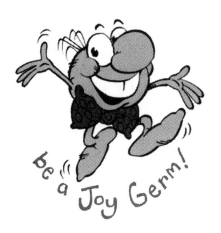

be a Joy Germ!

Tell people what you expect

Getting rid of visitors

Spot the visitor - jest for fun!

The telephone

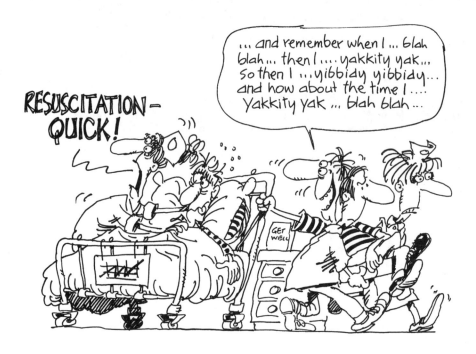

MOST PATIENTS ENJOY being visited in hospital. Even if you're very sick it is comforting to know that visitors are there. On the other hand, visitors can be tiring and stressful because you can't escape them. At least at home you can pretend to be out! In hospital there is nowhere to hide. The other problem is that some people don't know how to be helpful when they visit, especially if you have a life-threatening illness.

I chose a hospital two hours from home.
It guaranteed I'd be left alone.

Country Patient

TELL PEOPLE WHAT YOU EXPECT

Let your visitors know *when* you want them to visit and how *long* you want them to stay. It is also useful to know how to handle questions they may ask you. For example, when they ask "What's the problem?" don't feel obliged to tell them more than you are comfortable with. *You* have the choice. You can:

- Tell the truth.
- Be assertive and say "I really don't want to discuss it."

• Or have some fun by confusing them with unusual words or conditions... try 'Aprosexia', which is the inability to concentrate. Or 'Afflatus' - a sudden rush of divine inspiration. You can always say you have a 'Syndrome' - this sounds serious but could be anything. Another great reply is: "The doctors aren't really sure, but they say it's the most contagious thing they've ever come across!"

Some visitors will try to jolly you along with expressions like: "Cheer up, everything's going to be OK." Sometimes you will find this reassuring, but when you don't, say something like: "I know you're trying to make me feel better, John. But it makes me feel worse. I'd find it more helpful if you could..." - and then tell them!

GETTING RID OF VISITORS

As pleasant as visitors can be, even the ones you love, there will be times when you want to be left alone. We have seen too many patients stressed and exhausted at the end of visiting hours because they didn't want to risk offending their visitors by asking them to leave. As with house guests, sometimes you have to do more than merely hint to get them to leave. Here are some ideas:

• **Tell the nurses** that you are exhausted or upset by visitors and ask them to 'restrict' (use this word) visitor access to you. Then they'll put up a big sign saying something like 'Would visitors please report to the nurses' station before seeing patient'.

• **Be assertive.** *"Thank you for coming in, it's been good to hear about your plans for a holiday overseas. I need to be on my own now. I don't feel so good. Oh - and Tony, could you let the rest of the gang know I'm not quite up to visitors yet. Thanks. Bye."* **or** *"I'm expecting the nurses in any minute for some treatment, perhaps you'd better go now."*

• **Pretend** to be asleep, use a sleeping mask for effect.

• **Fake symptoms.** If all else fails: Try - diarrhoea (make several trips to the toilet), laryngitis (no speaking), writhing in pain.

Visitors were required to enter the ward via the main entrance and purchase a visitor's ticket for sixpence.

Isabel Gill, writing of her time as a nurse in 1938.

Spot the visitor - jest for fun!

The Stayer is a person without a life of their own. You can give hints, vomit, stop breathing, fake sleep, tell them you feel awful - but they *will not leave*.

The Remote Controller has developed the skill of commandeering the TV remote and punctuating the conversation with channel changes.

The Crowd: These visitors have no conversational difficulties at all - they talk only to each other.

The Bore depends on you to start and maintain the conversation. They add little to it. A human anaesthetic!

The Know-All need not be told about your operation. They already know more than you *and* your doctor.

The Doom-and-Gloomer spends his or her life collecting bad news. For every optimistic comment you make, they can produce an avalanche of misery in response.

The "When I was in hospital": There is only one thing worse than experiencing your own illness, and that is to be forced to learn all about someone else's - with accompanying gruesome details!

The Sanctimonious can be spotted before they open their mouth. They've got eyes like a basset hound's, slumped shoulders, drooping mouth and the appearance of a pall bearer. And all this for an ingrown toenail!

The Sticky Beak picks up your chart and says "You poor thing." Then, before you know it, they're questioning the nurses about your treatment.

The Boomer can be heard before you see them coming. No matter what you say to them confidentially, it is broadcast across the entire ward.

The Feeder arrives right on meal times with a voracious appetite for hospital food, especially yours! They bring you *their* favourite chocolates, open them and then scoff the lot before they leave. They love a "Fasting" sign.

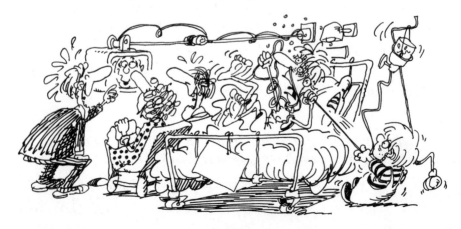

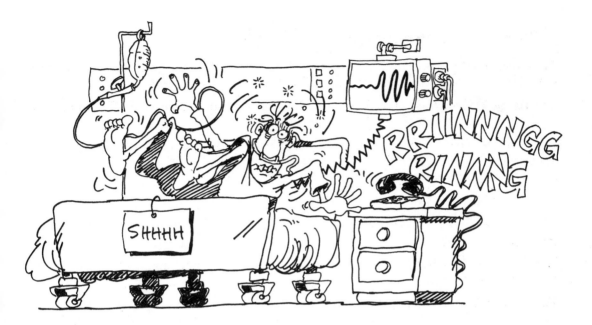

THE TELEPHONE

Picture the scene: You have had a difficult night, the pain is easing and you're in a deep sleep. Then the phone (next to your bed) rings. It doesn't matter who it is, this call may mean that you don't rest again that day.

What has been introduced to hospitals as a *service* to patients can sometimes *cause* stress and *slow down* recovery. As with visitors, you need to restrict telephone access if you're not well. If you love phone calls and feel better for them, make sure you ask for a private phone. But they *can* be tiring, so you may want the switchboard to put a 'Do not disturb' on your line or not have a phone at all.

> *As a hospital visitor, I see many things that cause stress. One of these is patients on the phone sorting out family problems at home.*
>
> Visitor

Patient: *Doctor, doctor, I think I swallowed a pillow.*
Doctor: *How do you feel?*
Patient: *A little down in the mouth.*

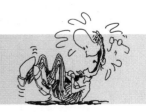

Your Notes

Chapter 5

Visiting Rites

– Helpful visiting

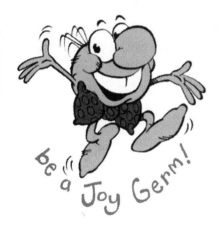

be a Joy Germ!

Be a welcome visitor

Bedside manners

Be a fun visitor

Gifts for patients

When the patient goes home

Special concerns

"I believe that how you visit a patient goes beyond friend visiting friend. It is about bringing strong medicine to the bedside. Inherent in the visit is actual involvement in the healing of the patient and the relief of suffering."

Dr Patch Adams

PATCH ADAMS HAS devoted much of his book *House Calls** to how visitors can be part of a 'healing team'. This is not always easy to do in a strange environment with a person who is sick. This is why so many people feel stressed at the very thought of being 'obliged' to visit someone in hospital, so they give up and resort to the standard bunch of flowers and awkward silences.

However, you can choose to be a thoughtful and creative visitor. Use the ideas in this chapter, and you'll be amazed at what you can achieve for the patient and for yourself.

BE A WELCOME VISITOR

Getting information

Appoint someone close to the patient - with the patient's consent - as an **'information person'** to make all the calls to the hospital. They can then let everyone else know what is going on either directly or through a **'telephone tree'**. This is because answering the phone for numerous enquiries can be very time-consuming and distracting for the nurses (and for the patient if they are taking phone calls).

Visiting hours

Visiting hours vary according to the type of hospital, the condition of the patient and your relationship to the patient. In a midwifery ward, for example, spouses and partners have priority. In critical care units, it is 'family only'. If you need to visit outside of visiting hours, phone the nurse manager ahead of time to explain your difficulty and ask him/her to help you out by 'allowing' a visit.

*Robert D Reed Publishers, 1998.

Check if the patient wants to see you

Telephone ahead and ask the staff to check with the patient whether they 'feel up to a visit' from you. This way you're more likely to know their real feelings as opposed to the patient's need to be 'nice'. Letting the patient know you're coming will increase their pleasure, because it's something to look forward to.

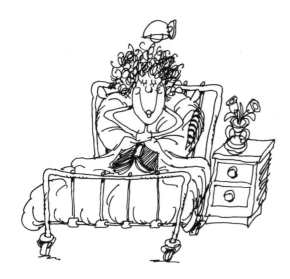

Patient before visitor

Know when to leave

Be prepared to spend some time - but know when to leave. Frequent, shorter visits can be more helpful than less frequent, longer ones.

Patient with visitor

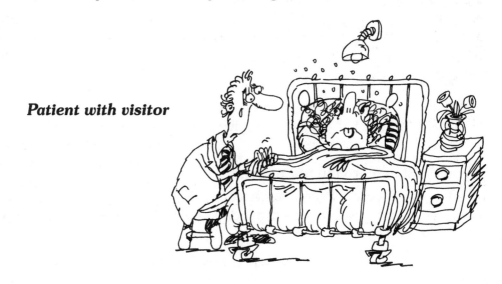

Time your visit

Patients are usually disorientated for a day after surgery or major treatments, so save your visit and your flowers until later. Some patients are embarrassed when friends see them looking their worst. At times you need to reduce your expectations of the patient in hospital. Illness, treatments and procedures cause some patients to be anxious, upset, irritable and impatient.

Be punctual. It's embarrassing to watch other patients' visitors arrive and there are none for you.

Patient

BEDSIDE MANNERS

- *"No, I brought those for you. All right then, I'll have just the one."* If you bring goodies for the patient let *them* have them.
- Don't walk over and talk to another patient and ignore yours.
- Avoid watching the television while you're talking - unless the patient joins you.
- Avoid giving advice. Listen attentively so the patient can work through *their* problems - not yours.
- Avoid staring at some poor soul in another bed.

Be sensitive

Listen, touch, laugh and cry! Patients are more likely to relax if you sit calmly, listen quietly, and accept their feelings. Ask "Would you like me to talk or just sit with you?" Sometimes the best thing you can do is put out your hand and touch the person.

Well-meaning comments like these are rarely helpful: "You'll be out of here in no time." "You've just got to be positive." "Don't worry, it's in God's hands."

If you can't see or visit the patient

- You could leave a loving message.
- Send a card or letter every other day - people love mail.
- Send flowers.
- Pray for the person.

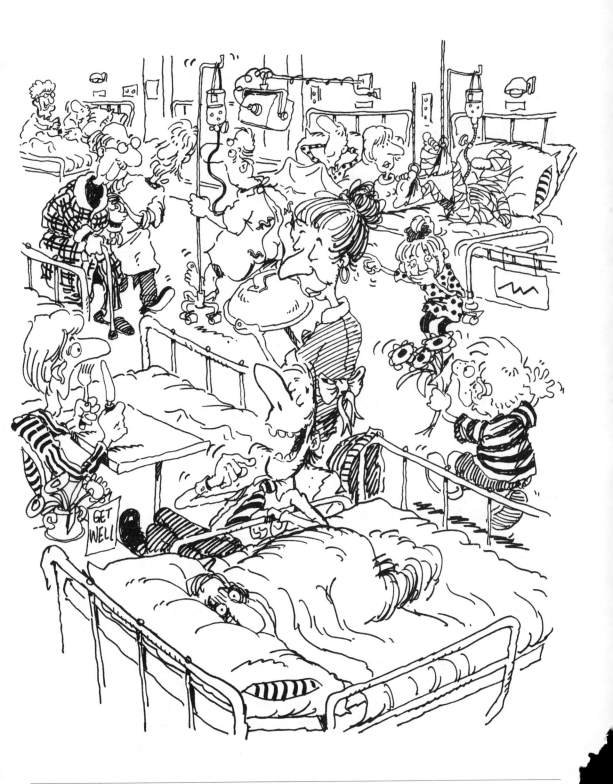

Help out

Call a family member and ask if you can do anything to help, eg transport, looking after children, chores or the shopping.

BE A FUN VISITOR

*The art of medicine consists of amusing the patient
while Nature cures the disease.*

Voltaire

This is where you have the chance to be creative. The good news is that what works outside a hospital works just as well inside. There is something to be said for the safety of numbers, so if you need to boost your confidence, find someone who will be wacky with you!

*I was amazed at how little I had to do as a clown. The
bright colours I was wearing and [my] big smile were such
a contrast to the drabness of the hospital. Patients just
loved to see me. Even if they had a thermometer in their
mouth, they still managed to smile.*

Hospital Clown

This doesn't mean you have to dress as a clown! There are a lot of things you could wear - bright clothes, or a funny tie, odd socks or a propeller hat can work wonders. Tell the patient you're the *Cheer Squad*. You'll find laughter will fill the silence, break down barriers and reduce the stress of being in hospital.

Sing

Everyone can sing. Some people are better at it than others, but willingness wins over talent. Involve the other patients and staff in singing a 'Get Well' ditty!

*One of the best lift rides I've ever had in a hospital was in St
Vincent's in Melbourne. I got the visitors and staff to sing the
Vegemite Jingle on the way up. Reluctant at first, they all
eventually joined in and we finished the ride laughing.*

Patricia

Play a musical instrument

Keep in mind that you are playing to cheer other people, it will help to reduce any nervousness you may have. You don't have to play perfectly.

Take games or cards to play together

We played cards or Uno... We would laugh and laugh because newer players would get confused when we started to change directions. We laughed so much that my sides hurt.

Patient

Fun attack

This is a surprise attack on an unsuspecting person or group of people. Make some funny hats out of newspapers; add balloons, a colourful garment and lollies to give to people and you're on your way.

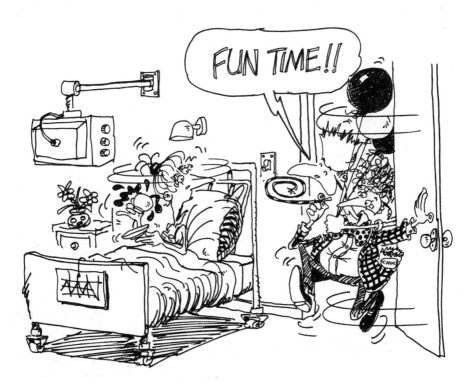

Visit the hospital 'laughter room'

Ask if the hospital has a 'laughter room' that you can visit with the patient. You'll find lots there to entertain you, including music, comedy videos, games, joke books, cartoons and dress-ups! (If the hospital doesn't have a 'laughter room', you may like to volunteer your services to help set one up!)

Visit the hospital garden

Most hospitals have a garden tucked away somewhere, or a public park nearby. Find a wheelchair and ask permission to take the patient into this place of natural healing. As a memento, take a photograph while you're there and as soon as possible bring it back to the patient, in a pleasant frame, to put on the locker.

Prepare a hospital surival kit

This is easy to organise if you think about the character of the patient, their lifestyle and their condition. Once you know what sorts of things would appeal, add to the standard items things like edible treats, ear plugs, cartoons and novelties. You can give this to a patient at any time and/or make up a special kit for when the patient goes home.

We took a survival kit to Pop. In it was a whistle to call for help, a badge [saying] 'Under Repair, Handle With Care', a smile on a lollipop stick, Minties, jokes and a safety pin for what we called 'Gown Gap-osis'. He loved it and showed it to all the other patients.

Visitor

Try to think of the hospital as a place of change and rest: The doctors get the change and the hospital gets the rest.

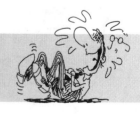

Humour is an antidote to stress

We mean positive, uplifting humour designed to raise the spirits of patients, visitors and staff. Just start with something you're comfortable doing, then become more daring!

Think of ways to get cartoons, jokes, funny videos and humour on tape and CD to your patient in hospital. For example:

- Wrap food in a cartoon.
- Send cartoons in the mail.
- Use a hospital VCR to show videos - invite other patients and visitors.
- Take in a personal cassette player and some humour tapes.
- Put jokes in envelopes, one to be opened each day the patient is in hospital.

A merry heart doeth good like a medicine; but a broken spirit drieth the bones.

Proverbs 17:22

GIFTS FOR PATIENTS

- Drinks. Spring or carbonated water will encourage fluid intake - check with the staff first.
- 'Thank You' cards or small-sized stationery, envelopes and stamps for the patient to use.
- Change for the public phone.
- Room spray, aromatherapy oil, small sprig of a fragrant flower (eg daphne) to freshen the air.
- A small bunch of flowers, in an inexpensive vase, will save space on the patient's locker.
- Food. Again, you'll need to check with the staff first. Favourite cooked meal, soup or scones. One or two pieces of fruit (instead of a basket of fruit which is often too green to eat), or a small container of chopped fruit. Chocolate biscuits. A range of herbal teas, or a thermos of favourite tea or coffee. Take a checked tablecloth to put on the bed and make it a picnic!
- Cheery magazines that are easy to read.
- A small bottle of scented massage oil.
- Photos.

WHEN THE PATIENT GOES HOME

They piled in [the hospital] with flowers and
gifts and when I got home I didn't have
anything. I wish they'd saved some flowers for
when I arrived home.

New mother

Have you ever had the experience of being in hospital as the centre of attention and as soon as you go home you are quickly forgotten? People think that because you are home you must be better and can take care of yourself. The truth is that more and more people are being sent home to *get* better!

There are a number a things that you can do to reduce stress for the person recovering their health at home. Here are a few suggestions; you'll soon think up others:

- Send flowers a couple of days *after* the patient has gone home.
- Take or send gifts of prepared food, especially soups and desserts.
- Take sandwiches - for both of you - when you visit.
- Organise some pre-paid home help for a week or so.
- Offer to take the patient's children for a day or two.
- Send letters and make phone calls on a regular basis for the first month at least.

SPECIAL CONCERNS

Visiting an unconscious patient

There is strong evidence that talking about everyday things, putting earphones on the patient so they can 'listen' to their favourite music and touching the patient, all add to healing. Accept that you may feel awkward doing this when you're not getting a response. *But do it anyway.*

I think every nurse should have a pet. This
would give them experience in talking and not
receiving a verbal response. Great training for
talking to an unconscious patient.

Nurse

If the patient is dying

*Dying is that process a few minutes before
death when the brain is deprived of oxygen;
everything else is living.*

Dr Patch Adams

We have included these words from Patch Adams to remind us all that people are either alive or dead. As long as they are alive, we must treat them that way.

This is because people who we consider to be 'dying' say that the worst part is being treated as if they are already dead. Most patients will want you to be a visitor who is cheerful, friendly and fun.

Remember funny stories to tell, share interesting articles, bring in a living plant, wear something wacky. Take your cue from the patient by asking a few 'open' questions to start with, such as "How do you feel about what's happening Jane?" "Would you like to talk about it?" or "What can I do while I'm with you today, to help you the most?"

Visiting the mentally ill

*Relax. Everyone is crazy to someone. If you're a people
watcher, then a mental hospital or patient can be a grand
privilege. Most mentally ill people are not dangerous; rather
they have unique ways of thinking and acting. Many are
first cousins to eccentrics and they are quite lovable.
So much of what is called 'mental illness' is really a
consequence of our troubled society - one that promotes
loneliness and conformity in a world whose gods are money
and power. Beware of people who think they are 'normal'.*

Dr Patch Adams

Thank you, Patch, for your reminder! If you embrace this message you are more likely to be flexible with, and less judgemental of, the mentally ill patient. But all of the ideas in this chapter can be useful, especially *being prepared to listen*.

Visiting children

Children are not miniature adults. They have special needs of their own when they are in hospital.

- If you are a parent or guardian, consider staying the night.
- When you leave, be sure to say when you'll come back again.
- If you can't come back when you promised, phone the hospital to give a message to your child.
- Take art materials - these allow your child to express thoughts and feelings.
- Read to your child or play stories on tape.
- Take puppets, or make puppets with your child, to help them express fears through the characters they create.

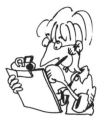

NOTES FOR STAFF

Think of ways visitors can be more active as part of the healing team - and let them know! You are welcome to make copies of this chapter and add your own ideas. When you see fun visitors in your area, give them some encouragement - and join in! Help visitors to feel more useful and less awkward in your ward or unit.

Did they really mean that?

From Doctors' dictating machines:

"According to witnesses, the patient was weaving down the street when he suddenly turned into an automobile."

"This man was brought in by his family because he is getting old and is losing his hearing, his memory and his urine."

"The patient was sent home in plaster."

"The pelvic examination will be done later on the floor."

"Father dies in his 90's of female trouble in his prostate and kidneys."

"The nursing home where the patient lives was noted to splutter, cough and run a fever."

Internet

Chapter 6

Kiss it better

– Pain relief

6

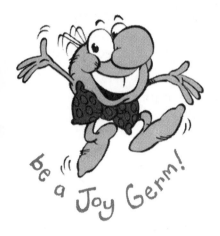

be a Joy Germ!

Pain is personal

Stress and pain

Comic relief

Mind over matter?

Relaxation/Meditation

Medications

More ideas

PAIN IS PERSONAL

"COME HERE DEAR, and I'll kiss it better." If you've ever heard these words, you will also remember how well this remedy worked. It was effective because it included attention from others, the reassurance of touch, and distraction from the injury. This is a perfect example of how the psychological component of pain can be managed.

One of the most important aspects of pain is to understand that *pain is personal.* No two people experience pain in the same way. The way you experience or perceive your pain will depend on both your psychological and physical states.

In addition to any medical problems, your psychological state is influenced by the type of person you are - your personality, how old you are, your culture, faith, family experiences and your gender. Your mood is also affected by your environment or what is happening around you.

Physical factors will also influence your response to pain. These include: nutrition, hydration (having enough fluids, particularly water), sleep, drugs, movement, posture, breathing, hormones and time of day.

Good news about pain relief

The personal and complex nature of pain means that there are many approaches to relieving it. They range from mind control to relaxation to intravenous narcotics - which all have their place. Our 'Kiss it better' example shows how simple some of these can be.

It is important to *keep an open mind* about pain relief, because no-one knows the best way of relieving your pain. You may have to be prepared to consider both conventional and complementary therapies, and try out a range of options.

The good news is that so much is known today about pain and how to relieve it. Some hospitals, for example, have pain control teams - comprising a range of health care professionals who work together to advise on the best approaches. You can access these *pain control clinics* by referral, as a patient in hospital, or as an outpatient.

The nurse who can smile when things go wrong is probably going off duty.

STRESS AND PAIN

Pain can be useful because it is a warning sign that something is wrong. But pain, if uncontrolled, can cause stress, slow your recovery and cause other problems.

Stress can also cause pain or make it worse - the stress that comes from worrying about your condition, a procedure, or how long it will be before you are well again. Even being anxious about the pain itself, (why it hurts, if it will ever stop hurting or if it will get worse), can exacerbate pain or your tolerance of it.

When you are in pain, you are less likely to move around, or do your deep breathing exercises or cough when necessary. You may also feel less like eating, drinking or going to the toilet. Pain can also make you feel depressed, 'down' and disheartened.

You should be able to deep breathe,
cough and sleep comfortably.

Pain Control Nurse

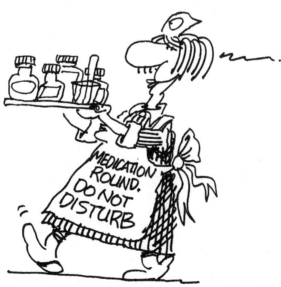

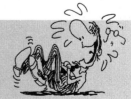

1st man: I woke up this morning and felt so bad that
I tried to kill myself by taking a hundred aspirins.
2nd man: Oh really, what happened?
1st man: After the first two, I felt better.

COMIC RELIEF

...ten minutes of solid belly laughter had an anaesthetic effect and would give me at least two hours of pain-free sleep.

Dr Norman Cousins

Norman Cousins was diagnosed with a spinal disease called *ankylosing spondylitis*, a painful degenerative disease with a one in 500 chance of recovery. Certainly nothing to laugh about! He started to think about the very stressful life he was living prior to the disease and wondered if it had anything to do with him getting sick. Deciding that it had, he was convinced that if stress and worry made him sick, then relaxation and laughter would get him well again.

What Norman Cousins did about this should give you great hope for your situation, and encourage you to use the ideas in this book. While a patient in hospital in 1976, he watched funny movies on a motion picture projector. He would have the nurse turn it on to get his belly laughter, then turn it off to get pain-free sleep. He had a collection of humour books that the nurses would sometimes read to him. He discovered to his delight, and to the surprise of staff, that laughter relieved his pain. Not only did it relieve pain, but laughter actually improved his condition, so that in conjunction with traditional medical treatment, he made a full recovery.

Endorphins

Medical research has discovered that when we laugh, especially belly-laughing, we secrete biochemicals known as *endorphins*. These are the body's natural narcotics, several hundred times stronger than morphine!

The other reason why laughter may control pain is that it relaxes muscles and reduces the stress associated with pain. Laughter also involves deeper breathing and improved circulation, which combine to reduce pain.

I don't feel like laughing!

For most people, laughing is the last thing they want to do when they are in pain. You may feel you have neither the strength nor the energy to find something funny, let alone start laughing. Even if you feel like this, still be prepared to surrender to the opportunity to laugh if it comes your way.

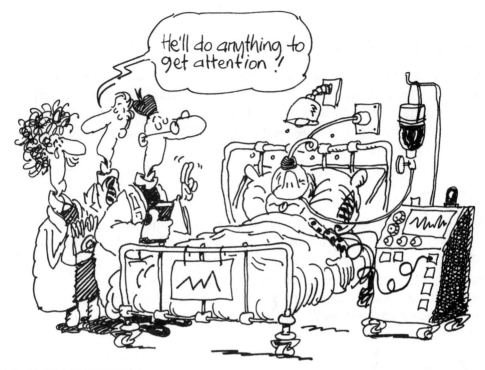

MIND OVER MATTER?

Pain is real. People do not *imagine* pain. But your mind does play a part in how you experience the pain, so mind control techniques must be considered. It may involve re-interpreting the pain - as did this patient recovering from a car accident:

> *What helped me was to say to myself, 'You don't have to feel the pain, just get on and mend it.' In fact, I called it 'discomfort' not 'pain', and it made a difference.*

Patient

The Placebo Effect

Medical researchers have conducted many studies that show the way the human mind converts thoughts and expectations into biochemical realities. Many people, when told what to expect from a medication's effect, will actually experience those effects even though the 'medication' is replaced by a pill containing nothing more than saline or sugar. This 'placebo effect' demonstrates the power of the mind to influence what goes on in your body, and shows the value of using this same power to control your pain.

RELAXATION TECHNIQUES

Pain can also be relieved by consciously relaxing each muscle group in your body. This also reduces stress and the muscle tension that can accompany the pain. Let your breathing *be slow and steady* and as you breathe out, let the tension go with the breath. Imagine breathing into your area of pain and as you breathe out, let the pain go with it.

MEDITATION

Meditation is a form of relaxation that calms the mind. It is a proven technique for relieving pain. In his book *You Can Conquer Cancer**, Ian Gawler has an excellent discussion of the physical and psychological causes of pain. Gawler offers a range of approaches to relieving pain, including meditation. He has used these methods personally and they have also been effective for thousands of people attending his workshops and residential programs.

Distraction

We have all used this technique at some time to stop a child from crying when they hurt themselves. It is a simple and powerful technique that gets your mind thinking about something other than your pain. This is why some of the relaxation tapes you use may have 'imagery' included. (Imagery is a way of taking the mind to a positive and relaxing place.) Other ways to distract your mind are included throughout this book and include music, books on tape, reading, laughter, television, friends and helping others.

Other non-drug pain relief options

To avoid some of the problems associated with pain relief drugs (addiction and altered mental states), especially in the long term, it is worth considering alternatives. These include hypnotherapy, acupuncture, physiotherapy treatments and local heat (hot water bottle/wheat bag).

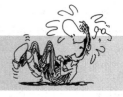

Patient: Doctor, I keep thinking that I'm a deck of cards!
Psychiatrist: Sit over there and I'll deal with you later.

*The Gawler Foundation, Phone Australia 03 5967 1730

MEDICATIONS OR 'PAIN KILLERS'

These are called 'analgesics' and can be administered by mouth (orally), on the skin, in a muscle (intramuscular), in a vein (intravenous), rectally, or into the spinal canal (epidural).

Oral medications

These can be in a liquid, tablet or capsule form. Most take 20-30 minutes to work and should be taken with plenty of water to make sure they enter the stomach and are absorbed as quickly as possible. As with all analgesics, most oral medications are best taken every four hours to maintain a constant level of the drug. (Always check the instructions).

My advice to patients is to ask for pain killers if you need them and ignore any lecture you may get on addiction.

Patient

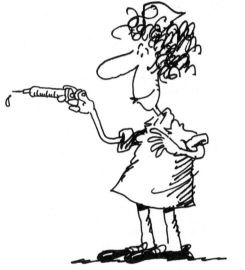

Injections

The most common injection is into the muscle of the leg or buttock. Make sure the nurses don't use the same spot for every injection, or the side you are most likely to want to lie on to sleep.

Patient Controlled Analgesia (PCA)

As an alternative to an injection into your muscle every four hours, self medication is sometimes used.

This involves pressing a button when you feel pain, and the pain-killing medication flows directly into your vein from a computerised pump. These pumps are useful for children who will often suffer in silence rather than have an injection! PCAs are portable and can be used at home.

An alternative is a continuous intravenous (into a vein) infusion, which is regulated by the nurses.

Epidural pain relief

A catheter (tube) is placed in the epidural space near the spinal cord and local anaesthetic drugs are pumped in to numb the nerves. This is most often used during labour in childbirth and for some operations, for example hysterectomy.

Bear in mind that the effect of an epidural can wear off quite quickly once the tube is removed, so if you are offered alternative pain relief at this stage - accept it!

Other ways of administering pain relief

A *patch* of medication applied to the skin, which is absorbed for up to three days. There are *also creams applied to the skin* for numbing prior to a needle insertion.

It is accepted practice to combine anti-inflammatory tablets (or suppositories) such as *Indocid* or *Naprosyn* with more common pain killers to reduce swelling and soreness.

MORE IDEAS FOR GETTING INVOLVED IN PAIN RELIEF

(See also Chapter 10)

- Be an informed patient. Ask questions and discuss pain control options *before* your operation or procedure.
- Let the nurses know when you first experience pain. Pain (anywhere) is the most common symptom of complications! The more pain builds, the higher the dose of pain killer you'll need and the pain will take longer to subside.
- Describe your pain as clearly as you can. You may even use a scale of one to ten to indicate its severity.
- Get involved in your pain management. Ask to see a doctor or nurse from a pain control service or clinic if you think you need more or different pain control.
- Ask to see a pharmacist to discuss the drugs you're using and the side effects. (Side effects such as nausea, vomiting, itching and constipation can be treated.)
- Let the nurses know if you feel light-headed or if you hallucinate while you're having continuous intravenous pain killing medication. It is usually a sign that the dose needs to be reduced. You should be pain-free without over-sedation!
- Make plans for managing your pain once you are home. District nurses usually have a good understanding of how to do this.

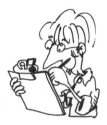

NOTES FOR STAFF

Dare we say it, but one of the drawbacks of working in hospitals is the risk that we become complacent about pain. It is easy to give routine analgesics, but it takes commitment and creativity to look for effective alternatives. Dr Norman Cousins' work in humour therapy and mind/body medicine is well worth reading. His books include *Anatomy of an Illness, The Healing Heart* and *Head First: The Biology of Hope.*

We should be encouraged by the placebo phenomenon. It is proof of the power of the mind and the value of including non-drug options for pain relief.

Did they really mean that?

From Doctors' dictating machines:

"Physical examination demonstrates a lady who was lying very pleasantly in bed."

"This unfortunate 45 year old woman has known me for about 8 years."

"Patient's abdomen is at war."

"Healthy appearing, decrepit 69 year old white female, mentally alert but forgetful."

"The patient was seen about four weeks ago by a physician with a urethral drip."

"The patient was admitted to hospital on the day of admission."

Internet

Your Notes

Chapter 7

'Drive thru' surgery

– Day surgery

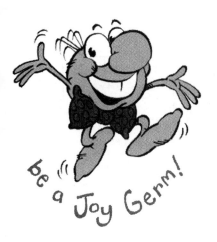

be a Joy Germ!

Recovery takes time

Choosing a day surgery centre

Get information

When to stop eating and drinking

Before the big day

After your operation

Rest

*I was in and out of hospital so fast,
I expected someone to ask
"Do you want fries with that?"*

Patient

EVERYTHING IS FAST these days. Fast food, fast dialling, fast banking, fast checkouts - and surgery is no exception. Medical science has given surgical procedures a smart new option - day surgery. It's slick, it's streamlined and it's here to stay. It means that hospitals can be run more economically and it caters for busy people who want a procedure done quickly.

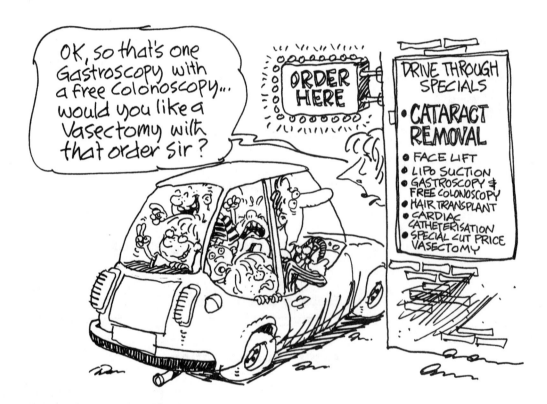

RECOVERY TAKES TIME

Advances in medical technology mean that it is easier to do many major procedures as *day surgery*. The biggest mistake made by people who are scheduled for day surgery is to think that because they are only in hospital for a few hours, their recovery will take a similar time.

What they don't appreciate is that the administration of an anaesthetic or sedative, to say nothing of an intrusive surgical procedure, are major sources of stress. It takes time to recover from all of this.

Surgery today is less invasive (more can be done with a smaller incision) and the procedure may be quick, but this does not mean that your recovery will be just as easy. **You didn't get sick in one day - you can't get better in one day!** Our advice is to ignore the clock on the wall and listen to your body clock.

Day surgery is a marathon not a sprint!

The other aspect of day surgery often overlooked is how stressful and tiring the whole event can be. It involves getting things in order at home, fasting, transport, checking in, waiting for any length of time, the procedure, recovery, checking out, transport home again. All the time not really knowing what is going to happen and when. We suggest you read other sections of this book and add these extra ideas so that you have a better understanding of what to expect.

The worst part of having day surgery was feeling like I was being processed, yet it was a very personal experience for me.

Patient

CHOOSING A DAY SURGERY CENTRE

Even though your surgeon may recommend a particular day surgery centre, you may have access to more than one, in which case you have a choice. You may even decide to look over a centre before you make up your mind. Day surgeries can be privately run as independent centres or attached to public and private hospitals.

Before having day surgery ask your doctor about the costs involved - not only for their own services, but for others including the anaesthetist, pathology tests and X-rays. As a public patient in a public hospital day surgery centre, all your costs should be met by the government.

In a private centre you may want to contact your health fund to make sure they have an arrangement with that centre and your doctor, and whether you will have 100% cover for charges.

GET INFORMATION

Make sure you get a copy of the day surgery centre's information booklet from your surgeon or the centre itself. Your surgeon may also have an operation information sheet available. Sometimes you have to ask for these. Also ask:

- What arrangements will be made if you are unable to go home the same day. **Day surgeries are not open at night.** This is less of a problem if the unit is attached to a hospital, but if it is not, you need to know.
- What time your operation is scheduled for (on the 'operating list') as opposed to the time you are meant to arrive at the Centre.
- How long you can expect to stay.

I wasn't as well as I thought I'd be after my operation. The doctor suggested I book into the hospital for the night. I agreed because I didn't think it would be fair on my niece to expect her to take on the responsibility of looking after me. I also felt more reassured - if something did go wrong the doctor was nearby.

Patient

WHEN TO STOP EATING AND DRINKING

You will need to ask what time you are meant to stop eating and stop drinking ('fasting') before your operation. If you are scheduled for a morning operation, then usually you fast from midnight onwards. For an afternoon operation, you usually fast from 6am. We recommend that you drink lots of water before this time and eat low fat food which is high in complex carbohydrates - oats, rice, wholemeal bread, bananas, pasta and potatoes.

Get some rest

I tried to get too much done before my operation. I didn't think there was much involved, so I worked right up to the last minute. I arrived at the Day Surgery Suite feeling stressed and worn out. Looking back, I don't think it helped my recovery.

Patient

That patient says it all. Plan to finish your work at least a day ahead of the operation so you can relax. We suggest some uplifting reading, videos or movies. Some laughter medicine is excellent.

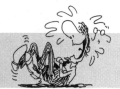

Hospitals never give you the one thing that you need - safety pins for the back of your gown.

Let your surgeon know if you have a cold

Having a cold may complicate your anaesthetic, so if you have any sign of a cold the day before (or the day of) your operation, let the surgeon know. These signs include a runny nose, a temperature or a sore throat. The surgeon will discuss with you whether it may be best to postpone your operation until you are well again.

OTHER THINGS TO DO BEFORE THE BIG DAY

- You will need to complete a **registration form** or similar and send it to the day surgery centre - your surgeon's staff may arrange this for you.

- **Phone the unit** the day before to confirm your arrival time - this is usually an hour before your procedure.

- **Wear light, comfortable clothing** - you will put this in a locker before you have your operation.

- **Take a few toiletries,** such a toothbrush and comb, etc to freshen up before you leave.

- **Leave valuables and jewellery at home** - if you want to wear a ring during the procedure, ask for it to be taped.

- **Make-up and nail polish** is best not worn. This is for reasons of hygiene and also because the anaesthetist will want to see the true colour of your face and nail beds.

- **Bring any medications** that you are taking, so they can be reviewed in the light of your post-operative requirements.

- **Take in** your personal cassette or CD player, relaxation music, and a favourite book on audiotape.

While I was on the trolley waiting I listened to comedy on my [personal cassette]. It was great to laugh before my operation. It certainly got my mind off things and I was more relaxed.

Patient

Prepare for a marathon day

If I had known it was going to take so long, I would have brought a picnic basket and gone to the park!

Relative

Make sure your friend or family member accompanying you brings something to eat and drink as well as something to read while they wait. A mobile phone is ideal for this sort of day and is worth borrowing if you do not have one of your own.

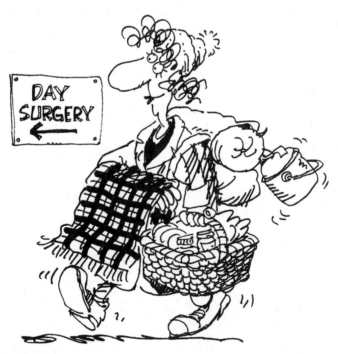

You cannot drive yourself home after day surgery

All surgical procedures involve sedation or an anaesthetic. Even though you may feel perfectly alright, it is quite a different matter when you try to concentrate and make decisions. For the next 12-24 hours, avoid driving, operating machinery or doing anything that requires you to be alert and co-ordinated. Have your family call for you at the day surgery unit. If the person picking you up is not driving, they may consider a taxi, or if finances permit, a limousine hire car for a smoother and more predictable ride home.

AFTER YOUR OPERATION

- **Start drinking water.** It is much better for you to start drinking sparkling or still spring water than to have a cup of tea. You need to rehydrate as soon as possible after a fasting period, and tea and coffee are dehydrating and unsuitable at this time.

- **Eat light food.** Eat food that is low in fat and high in complex carbohydrates. Continue this for at least 24 hours.

- **Make sure you know exactly what to do when you get home.** You may need to have instructions written down.

- **Know when and how to call your surgeon.** Most surgeons specify that they are to be called if *anything* untoward occurs. You need to know what that means and call them if you are worried. If your surgeon is not on call you need to know who else to call - perhaps a locum medical service. Keep the number handy.

- **You can arrange for a district nurse to call** each day (usually for a modest fee).

- **Don't drink alcohol** after your procedure because it will increase the anaesthetic/sedative effect.

- **Arrange and keep a follow-up appointment with your surgeon.**

Remember there are a few things you should give up while recuperating. Like cleaning, ironing, cooking, laundry, etc

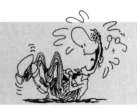

REST - even if you think you don't need it

To give your body a chance to heal, you should rest for at least 12-24 hours after your procedure - even if you feel 'fine'. Arrange for someone to be at home with you during this time and close by when you are standing and walking. You never know when your condition could change without notice.

Thereafter, take the time you need to be quite well. If you go back to work too soon, the stress involved will compromise your full recovery.

NOTES FOR STAFF

It is a real challenge for any day surgery centre to balance its need for speed and efficiency with the patient's need for information and to feel important. Patients feel important when they are received warmly at Reception, their name is used, their privacy is ensured and they are treated as intelligent adults. These things are all easy to do.

When you don't have details of the patient's home situation, then you have to provide enough information so that they (or their carers) can work things out for themselves - especially getting a doctor or organising for home nursing.

Read this book for more ideas on how to take the stress out of being in a day surgery centre for you and your patients.

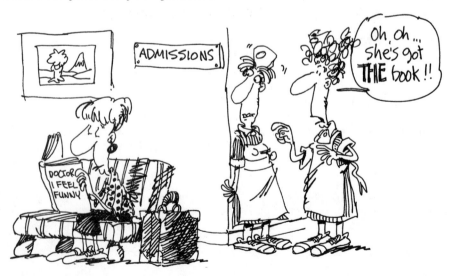

Chapter 8

Get well soon 8
– The healing power of the mind

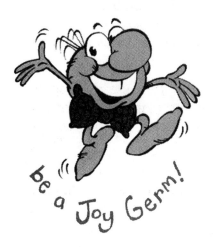

be a Joy Germ!

How are you today?

The mind/body connection

Mood changes

If you think you can, you can

Choose positive thoughts

Watch your language!

Feeling guilty?

Fed up?

Never lose hope

HOW ARE YOU TODAY?

THIS IS A true story. It happened some years ago in a Melbourne hospital:

> *As she was waiting for the trolley to take her to the operating theatre to have radical surgery that would change her life for ever, the woman was thinking her life was over. There was nothing to live for now. But then she saw a bunch of balloons coming towards her. In fact, they were coming for her. Attached to the trolley to take her to the operating theatre was a big bunch of balloons. There was also a smiling porter and, sitting on the trolley, a little bear dressed in an operating theatre gown. At that moment, the woman said, she realised that there would be a life for her after surgery. The porter explained that the balloons were to celebrate her trip to the operating theatre and her road to recovery.*

There is no question that the change in the way that woman felt about her future would have had a positive impact on her response to surgery. The story also encourages us to look at hospitals as wonderful places where people come together with their talents, skills and caring to promote healing and recovery. A *celebration*.

Being in hospital is not always easy. It is a major lifestyle adjustment to leave your family and friends, your pets, the garden, your hobbies and your job. It is normal to be concerned about how the outcome of your stay in hospital will affect your future. You may feel stressed, anxious, fearful or even angry.

On the other hand, you may be glad to be in hospital and have a sense of relief that something is being done. Some people appreciate the rest and the chance to take stock of their lives. They expect to have a laugh and new experiences, meet new friends, and enjoy being the centre of attention for a while. If this is your situation, you are likely to feel happy, relaxed and joyful.

It is important to remember that *everyone feels differently about being in hospital and that all feelings are acceptable.* Feelings are neither good nor bad, they just *are*.

One of the healthiest things a man can have up his sleeve is a funny bone.

THE MIND/BODY CONNECTION

The mind's greatest impact is felt on the *immune system*. Your immune system is the part of your body which fights disease and gets you well again; it defends you against invading viruses and bacteria which may cause infections and disease.

When you're happy your body knows it. When you're sad and feel hopeless or stressed, your body also knows it. Studies have shown that the immune system functions best in response to positive feelings, like *love, hope, the will to live, confidence, a sense of purpose, forgiveness, faith* and *joy*.

In contrast, negative feelings - such as *fear, panic, guilt, anger, resentment, hate, despair, helplessness, sadness, blame* and *remorse* - have the opposite effect and tend to depress the function of the immune system.

MOOD CHANGES

Your mood, the way you feel, is influenced by many things. Physical factors have more impact than people realise. These include what food you have eaten and when you last ate, whether you're hydrated (have had enough water), how much sleep you've had, what time of day it is, your hormones, how much exercise you've had, the air you're breathing, and your posture or position. We can add to these factors your medical condition and any drugs or treatment you're having.

There are also environmental factors such as the type of room you're in, its colours, furnishings, view, occupants and noise level. Then there are the people you see, fragrances, hugs, pets, music, clothes, singing, faith, dancing, massage, and so on. All of these have an impact on your mood.

This book is designed to help you to see how you can change the way you feel by changing aspects of your environment, to feel better and less stressed. There will, however, be times when you have to put up with less-than-ideal conditions; you'll find yourself in situations for which you are responsible and over which you have no control.

When this happens, you need to have strategies for managing the way you feel by *choosing* the way you look at things.

It's not what happens to you, it's how you take it that counts!

IF YOU THINK YOU CAN, YOU CAN

You always have a choice in the way you choose to feel about something. This choice is based on the thoughts you think, the beliefs you hold, and the way you speak to yourself. Most people don't pay much attention to what they think about, nor where those thoughts sprang from. We talk to ourselves all day long and half the night. This 'self talk' is at a speed of around 500 words per minute and we generate about 50,000 thoughts every 24 hours. Thoughts about life, the world, our feelings, problems and other people. These are the basis for our reality.

The problem with most of these thoughts is that they are negative.
Do these sound familiar?

"I bet no-one visits today."
"That doctor doesn't know what he's doing - I like my old doctor better."
"I hate the food."
"I bet nobody's watering my garden."
"Here they are - late again."
"I'm not looking forward to this."
"I bet I'll be awake all night again."
"The nurses hate me."

It is important to know that you have a *choice* in the thoughts you think. This is useful when you find yourself in a situation over which you don't have control.

What influences our thinking

We live in a negative world. The media, for example, celebrates pain. It doesn't take long to feel 'down' if you read a newspaper, or listen to the news on radio or watch it on television. Song lyrics can be depressing. The attitudes of people around us, movies, shows on television and our politicians don't exactly fill us with hope and optimism!

Thoughts are important because they cause you to feel a certain way and these feelings can be negative and cause stress, or positive and promote healing. This doesn't mean that just thinking positive thoughts will cure you - but it is proving to be an influencing factor.

So be careful what you put into your mind, especially when you are sick or your resources are low. Read uplifting material, talk to happy people and share in good news. When possible, limit your exposure to depressing people, and to books, news and shows which can bring on 'the blues'. *When it comes to health, it's the thought that counts.*

I watched John Wayne movies on television and was reminded of how tough he was. Then when I was having a difficult time of things, I said to myself 'How would John Wayne react to this?' Then I did the same.

Pitta Laungani as a patient

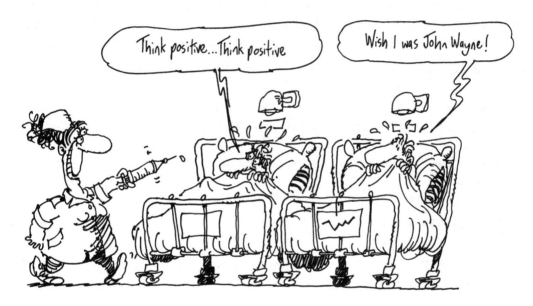

CHOOSE POSITIVE THOUGHTS

It's as simple as ABC to change your thoughts:

A - Acknowledge the thoughts you're thinking, whatever they are

B - Breathe deeply and slowly

C - Change your thoughts, say to yourself, over and over: *I am in good hands. My body knows what to do and I will be well again.*

Here are some examples of positive thoughts you can choose:

"I've handled tough times before, and I can handle this one."
"I'm so lucky to have these skilled people around me."
"Things could be worse."
"I know my body can heal itself."
"It may hurt but I can handle it."
"The nurses love me."

WATCH YOUR LANGUAGE!

When you stop to think about it, we say the strangest things. When things are going well, we seem to want them to end - we say, "It's too good to last." Yet, when things are going badly, we seem to want more of it, and we say, "It always comes in threes."

The way we talk to ourselves and to other people is mostly from habit and we don't always stop to think about it. Yet the words you use to describe an experience will become your experience. Like thoughts, the words you choose can have an impact on the way you feel and how well you respond to treatment. So choose your words carefully.

For example, when you are about to have a potentially painful procedure such as an injection, instead of saying, "I bet this will hurt," take a deep, relaxing breath and say to yourself, "I can handle this," or "I've handled tough times before and I can handle this one." Change the words and you can change the way you feel about it.

Here are some more ideas:

Instead of....	Say....
Heart attack	*Little problem with my heart*
Hot flushes	*Power surges*
Problem	*Challenge*
Furious	*Disenchanted*
Nervous	*Excited*
Can't sleep	*Awake*
Depressed	*A little bit down*
Sick	*Biologically challenged*
Dying	*Living*
Grumpy	*Not myself*

Something that helped me was to send love to the parts of my body that needed it most. So many times I heard people refer to their 'bad' leg or their 'bad' arm. My right leg was smashed to pieces in the accident, but it came through. I called it my 'good' leg and I'm sure it made a difference.

Patient

The way you respond to the everyday question **"How are you?"** will have a major impact on the way you feel. There will be times when you feel awful and it's all right to say that. At other times - when you want to cheer yourself, visitors or staff - you could try one of these:

- "fantastic"
- "full of beans"
- "unstoppable"
- "smashing"
- "terrific"
- "improving"

Or if you're none of these, say "Fine, if you don't want details."

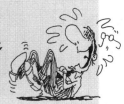

Someone told us at a seminar one day that his mother had moved from New Zealand to live in the United States. Everywhere she went she was told "Have a nice day." In the end she got sick of hearing this, so whenever someone said it to her, she would reply "Thank you, but I've made other arrangements!"

Patricia.

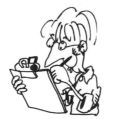

NOTES FOR STAFF

The way you choose to talk to yourself has a lot to do with how you feel at work each day. For example, "We're going to be busy today. I hate it when we're busy." This could be, "We're going to be busy today. I can handle it." Instead of responding to beepers and telephones with, "Who is it now? I'll never get my work done," choose, "That's my job." Let's face it, if the phones and beepers stop, you probably won't have a job.

Be careful with the words you use to talk to patients and visitors. Too many health care professionals worry about giving false hope - to us, it is far better than false fear!

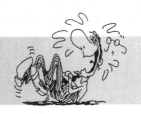

I said to myself: "Self," I said, "Cheer up. Things could get worse." So I cheered up and, sure enough, things got worse.

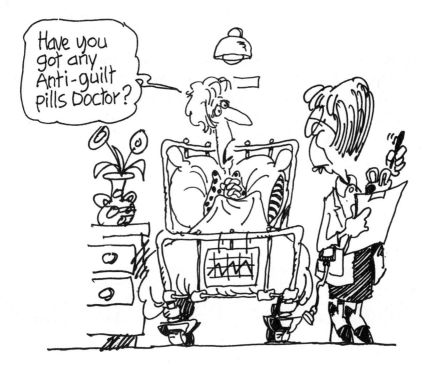

FEELING GUILTY?

Whether you are a patient or a visitor, you *may* be experiencing guilt. Do any of these thoughts sound familiar?

"If I'm the one who's sick, why do I feel so guilty? I didn't ask to get sick. What have I done to deserve this?"

"I wish I hadn't said anything, I feel really guilty now."

"I really should go home to look after the kids."

"I'd better make the effort to visit, otherwise I'll just be home feeling guilty."

You are not alone if you feel guilty. Mothers feel guilty about asking to stay in hospital a little longer. Older people can feel they are a burden on their families - and feel guilty. Parents can feel guilty about their child's illness or accident. Staff feel guilty because they make mistakes or forget to do things. Patients feel guilty for having accidents or getting sick. A new mother can feel guilty because she is not breastfeeding. Patients feel guilty if the treatment isn't working for them. Others feel guilty because they take up the time of the staff.

I felt guilty about feeling guilty.

Mother

Guilt is a feeling that comes from thinking that we *should* be doing something or *should not* be doing it. Sometimes we base these ideas on our standards, but more often they are influenced by what we have heard from other people, especially those with authority in our lives. We find ourselves doing things (or not doing them) and feeling guilty because we worry what other people will think of us.

One way to reduce the stress associated with guilt, is to know that you have the power to *choose not to feel guilty.* It's been our experience that when people value themselves, or feel good about themselves, they are less likely to feel guilty when they don't please others.

For example, next time you are about to use the word 'should', replace it with 'could' and note how much better you feel.

It may also mean changing the way you look at things, setting your own standards and *not worrying about what other people think of you.* It sounds tough, but it can be done. *No one can make you feel guilty without your permission.*

> *Most people are doing the best they can, given what they know and understand. If they knew more or understood more, they may do things differently. Including you.*
>
> Louise Hay

Accept your weaknesses and acknowledge your strengths

> *What other people think of you is none of your business.*
> Andrew Mathews

Know that you can't be like everyone else, because you're not them! *You are unique.* Unique in your response to life's challenges, the way you see things, your illness, your response to treatment, the way you look after someone else, your healing process, what makes you comfortable, and so on.

> *Everyone makes mistakes. When you make a mistake, separate the mistake, or your actions, from who you are. Say to yourself: 'That was a dumb thing to do, but I am not dumb.'*
>
> Patricia

Be kind to yourself

"I'll never forgive myself," or "If only..." are phrases that will keep you in the past and make you feel guilty. Instead, try saying "I'm only human. I forgive myself and will do what needs to be done," or, "Next time I will..."

Accept responsibility for what happened (if you're at fault), let it go, then deal with the consequences in a constructive way. If you stay stuck in the past, it will sap the energy you need to deal with the present and the future.

FED UP?

*During those dark days I learned that suffering
need not destroy.*

Terry Waite (Held hostage for 1763 days in the Middle East)

You know when you are fed up. You question the value of the treatment you are having and the competence of the people giving it to you. Your friends try to be helpful by relating their near-death experiences and what worked for them. They give you names of people they swear will do a better job than those you have looking after you. In the end, you still feel awful - and now have nagging doubts and feelings of despair.

You wonder if you will ever be right again. You think you will have the pain forever, that it will never go. You think of all the things you would like to be doing and know you cannot do them. You start to think of what life could be like if you never get well again.

These and similar thoughts are common for most people during their stay in hospital and once they go home, especially if their recovery is prolonged. If you are feeling 'fed up', be reassured that it is a *natural and normal* way to feel. The worst thing you can do is start to feel guilty for feeling this way!

Being defeated is often a temporary condition; giving up is what makes it permanent.

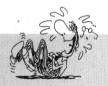

Psychiatrist's advertisement: Satisfaction guaranteed or your mania back!

Healing takes time

Keep in mind that healing and recovery do not necessarily occur in a straight line. Think of it as standing in the middle of a see-saw. Sometimes you go up, and sometimes you go down. Gradually, with recovery, you start to stay up for longer than you are down. The important thing is to accept that some days are just for surviving, and not to give up.

In our experience, most people underestimate just how long it takes to heal. Medical technology assists healing but, in the end, nature must cure. It is important to recognise the signs of the healing process, even if they are small. These may include: staying awake longer during the day, walking a few extra steps, eating something extra, getting a little more pain-free sleep, a happier hour, an improved blood test or X-ray, or needing fewer pain killers.

NEVER LOSE HOPE

Getting well is not the only goal. Even more important is learning to live without fear, to be at peace with life, and ultimately death.

Dr. Bernie Siegel in *Love, Medicine and Miracles*.

It can be tempting sometimes to prepare ourselves for the worst rather than be let down by false hope. But all the information available points to the power of hope in influencing the outcome of disease and treatment. In his book,* Dr Norman Cousins, expresses his doubt that anyone knows enough to deny hope:

I have seen too many cases these past ten years when death predictions were delivered from high professional station only to be gloriously refuted by patients for reasons having less to do with tangible biology than with the human spirit, admittedly a vague term but one that may well be the greatest force of all within the human arsenal.

(*Head First*, pp 65,66)

*Head First: The Biology of Hope and the Healing Power of the Human Spirit.
Penguin Books 1990

After many years spent with patients facing life-threatening illnesses, Dr Cousins advised them to *accept* the diagnosis and the treatment, but *challenge the verdict that is meant to go with it.*

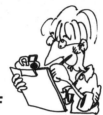

NOTES FOR STAFF

[Reassurance] is not a Pollyanna concoction aimed at deception. It is not a verbal tranquilizer for creating a mood or synthetic calm. It is a way of putting the human spirit to work, a way of respecting the desire of a patient to confront a new challenge; a way of summoning all one's strength and resources in the most important fight of one's life.

(*Head First*, pp 66)

We recommend any of the books written by Dr Bernie Siegel, especially *Love, Medicine and Miracles.** Also those written by Dr Norman Cousins, especially *Head First.* Their books are informative, inspirational and down-to-earth: a rare combination!

*Arrow Books 1986

Chapter 9

The hospital, faith and fear

– Dr Francis Macnab

Written for this book by Dr Francis Macnab who is a Psychologist and Psychotherapist. He is the Executive Director of the Cairnmillar Institute, Chairman of The Australian Foundation for Aftermath Reactions to Trauma and Executive Minister of St Michael's Uniting Church, Melbourne.

THE HOSPITAL, FAITH AND FEAR

The door closed. What did she say? "Put this white gown on back-to-front and tie it at the back."

All clothes off. This bare little space; I start to realise I am so bare in this little space. No cords on the gown to tie it. Will I ask for another? No - they will think I'm a nuisance. I climb up onto the high bed. I stare at the ceiling. I know I am alone. Alone in the room. Alone as I prepare for this procedure that will tell me I have a huge tumour in my stomach. This is what I fear.

Before I left home the three girls all went off to school. Not one of them showed the slightest hint that they had a worry about their mother going into hospital today. I'm 46. This is the day when everything could change. Surgery, chemo, checkups. Two of my friends have been through it and one of them is already dead. Her husband quickly married again. I wonder if David will marry again. He's only 47.

My mother is a bagful of worry about me. My father did not say much, but I could see the burden of grief already on his face.

Oh God, help me! God!

I haven't thought about God since the day I was married. (Or was it the day we decided not to send our eldest to Sunday School?)

If there is ever a time when a person feels the need for God it is in a room like this, lying in a hospital gown that has no cords at the back. I stifle a nervous laugh and close my eyes.

I think I want to say a prayer. For the three girls. They are so young. And for David - that his next wife will not be as good as me! I laugh again. What a prayer - and I'm a long way from being dead.

Nobody comes. They purposely leave you alone to agonise; or maybe they want me to realise what this whole trip means.

In the quietness, I get the message: I am alone. I need this quietness to give me a little bit of courage. I breathe slower. It is as if the angels are waiting for me. I interrupt myself with another small laugh - who believes in angels?

The walls of this room seem to be friendlier now. They are like a gentle blanket wrapping around me. I notice that I have stopped trembling.

Oh God, help me.

I feel a strength and a quietness inside me. There is some kind of hope around me. I feel more at peace than I have for weeks. God, what a good thing silence can be.

The door seems to crash open. A nurse, and the anaesthetist. He says, "All ready?" He probably says that to everybody, meaning, "Have we tied the cords at the back of the gown?" But for me, those words mean something totally different.

I'm ready.

They roll me onto their trolley, and just before they push and pull me through the door, I look back over my head at the bare walls of that room.

I wonder how many people speak to God in that room? How many people in their loneliest moments feel a presence that steadies them? We may not all call it 'God', but that sense of being held or encouraged gives each one of us the strength to say, "I'm ready," no matter what the outcome or the pathway ahead.

Three hours later the surgeon was standing at my bedside. It took me a few moments to get my eyes into focus. I knew by his face what he was about to say. I was 'ready' for it. I was quickly on an unknown pathway with the shadow of death following me.

At the same time, I was on another pathway where I began to discover new things about myself and new things about life. I discovered my own new faith. Faith, I realised, was to hold onto hope that whatever was going to happen to me, there was something deeper. It was like those walls of the room, wrapping around me, and telling me that this was the strength to let go of all my anxieties and be at peace. I might not get better, but this inner peace and strength - was it faith? - would console me and heal me at that deeper level.

David came to see me. He said he picked up a card in the hospital foyer. He would leave it with me to read later. What a strange coincidence! It read - 'Though I walk through the valley of the shadow of death, I will fear no evil - Your rod and Your staff they comfort me.'

Your Notes

A dog and me and TLC

– Comfort ideas

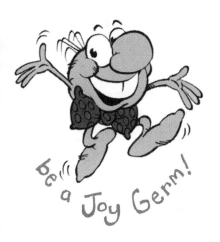

be a Joy Germ!

A dog
_____

TLC (Tender Loving Care)
_____

Massage
_____

Aromatherapy
_____

Music
_____

Relaxation
_____

Nature
_____

Other comforts
_____

A DOG

THERE WAS A knock on the door of the patient's room. He had a splitting headache and dreaded the idea of more blood tests or procedures. "Come in," was what the patient murmured, but he really wanted to say "Go away." When the door opened, it was a smiling nurse who asked, "Do you feel well enough to have a dog visit?" The patient nodded.

In walked a beautiful golden Labrador with his owner. The nurse prepared for the visit by putting a drawsheet on the bed and then the owner lifted the dog on to it. At once the patient smiled and started stroking the dog, the dog responded by nuzzling against him. During this time, the patient and owner talked about dogs, especially the patient's own dog which was at home.

For 20 minutes the patient stroked the dog. At the end of the visit, the patient said his headache had lifted and he was starting to feel better. He thanked the owner and asked if he the dog could visit him again the next day. The patient was left smiling and relaxed.

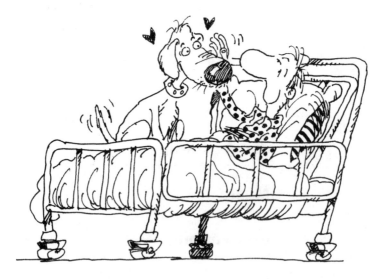

Fantasy?

This is a true story which we had the privilege of seeing for ourselves in Huntington Memorial Hospital in California. It is an 800 bed, acute teaching hospital that has a pet therapy program for patients. At the time of our visit, the program had 30 dogs (many breeds) and their owners from the local community who volunteered a number of hours each week to the hospital.

Pets and healing

Pets are a natural and effective way to take the stress out of being in hospital. It is now scientifically proven that when you stroke an animal that you like, your blood pressure and pulse lower and you feel more relaxed. Pets can also provide a wonderful distraction from pain and procedures.

What you can do

If your hospital has a pet visiting program (sometimes known as 'Pets-As-Therapy'), ask for a visit. If they don't have a program, then send a note to the hospital manager suggesting that they initiate one. Ask the staff if your pet can be brought in from home to visit you. If the pet cannot come to your bedside, perhaps you could see the pet in a different area. Another idea is to have photos of your pets enlarged on a photocopier and put them around your bedside.

When I was in hospital, what I missed most was my pet goats. To my surprise one day, my friends smuggled them into the hospital to see me. It gave me a real lift.

Patient

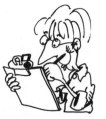

NOTES FOR STAFF

What we did not expect to discover on the 'dog round' we joined was the impact the dogs had on the *staff*. On seeing a dog, the staff member would stop, smile and pat the dog. A great way to reduce stress for staff as well as patients. The dogs visited all areas including high dependency. **Why not set up your own pet program?** Contact Huntington Memorial Hospital in California* to buy a manual on how to go about establishing a Pets As Therapy (PAT) program.

*100 West California Blvd. Pasadena 91109 USA

TLC - Tender Loving Care

Your hospital stay can be transformed with punctuations of comfort. It will take a little thought and creativity (and perhaps effort on someone's part), but it is worth it. Our TLC ideas take the stress out of being in hospital by providing comfort; they promote healing and wellness.

In considering these ideas, keep in mind that whatever you decide to use only has to work for you and does not have to make sense to anyone else! The exception, of course, is any action considered by medical opinion to compromise your health and recovery. Any disapproval based on personal opinion which is not based on scientific proof nor experience, should be questioned. You have a right to try things that may enhance your comfort, and your body's own healing system. They will, in turn, enhance the effectiveness of your medical treatment.

MASSAGE

I was in hospital when my family was away. Once I started to feel better, I asked for a massage - not only because I was on a hard mattress cover, but because I missed the comfort of touch from another human being.

Patient

If you have ever had a massage, you will not need to be convinced of the benefits. Massage is now considered to be a powerful healer because it can improve your circulation, relax tired and tense muscles, lower your blood pressure, reduce pain and stimulate your immune system. Massage can also improve your mental state. The simple act of *touching* lets you know that you are not alone and is an indispensable part of the healing process.

Massage need not be complicated

Most people can give a simple massage to your hands, feet and legs. You can use a handcream or massage oils or lotions which may contain essential oils to refresh and ease tense muscles. (Massage is also recommended for unconscious patients for both physical and mental benefits.)

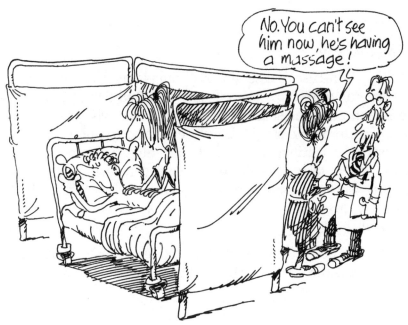

Massage Therapist

Some enlightened hospitals have massage therapists on staff and/or encourage nurses to learn massage. Alternatively, you could ask for a massage therapist in private practice to come into the hospital to give you a massage. Ask for this service or consult your telephone directory for clinical masseurs who are prepared to visit.

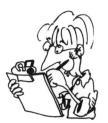

NOTES FOR STAFF

Some hospitals have now introduced massage for staff as well as patients. In some hospitals the cost is subsidised by the hospital in the interests of reducing stress and saving on sick leave costs.

Consider making this suggestion where you work. This will enhance awareness of the value of massage for staff and for patients. As long as it is considered an 'optional extra', there will never be enough time to include massage as part of patient care.

Meanwhile, remember to use touch in your nursing care - holding the patient's hand, touching the forearm and supporting the patient's forehead when they're vomiting. Try to find ways to include a simple hand or foot massage in the care of your patients - even a few minutes can make all the difference.

TLC - Aromatherapy

Aromatherapy is the use of essential oils from plants to refresh and to relax, and to improve general wellbeing. The effect is achieved through our sense of smell and absorption through the skin. For example, some oils - such as lavender and sandalwood - can promote sleep. Lavender is also useful to relieve headaches. Aromatherapy* uses a range of products including bath and massage oils and body lotions. As a safer alternative to using candle burners (especially near oxygen outlets), electric aromatherapy stones are available from pharmacies. Or simply put a few drops of the appropriate oil on a cotton wool ball and place it inside the pillow case.

Essential oils are powerful in their effect and require informed use, particularly if you are pregnant (first trimester), or have a medical condition such as high blood pressure or epilepsy.

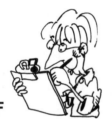

NOTES FOR STAFF

Have you ever been caught in a lift with someone wearing a powerful *perfume* or *aftershave?* It is such a relief when the doors open and you can escape. Keep in mind that patients can't escape your perfume or aftershave. Even a fragrance you consider subtle may not be subtle for a patient. People who are sick have a lowered tolerance to perfumes. Avoid wearing perfume or aftershave in patient areas.

TLC - Music

Appropriately selected music can make you feel less stressed and more relaxed. Music can also divert your thoughts to other places to recall happy memories, so you can enjoy them all over again. Take care in selecting your music - it has the potential for both pleasant and unpleasant reactions.

Works by Bach feature amongst the most relaxing classical music and there is a wide range of contemporary relaxation music available.

* The Body Shop has a wide range of aromatherapy products and information about their safe use.
Mail order. Phone Australia 03 9565 0520.

TLC - Relaxation

Although it is normal to feel stressed at times when you are in hospital, your body heals best when you are relaxed. You can learn to consciously relax your body whenever you feel anxious or tense. The starting point is always with your breathing. Breathe slow and steady and as you breathe in, feel the cool air coming in through your nose (or mouth) and warm air coming out.

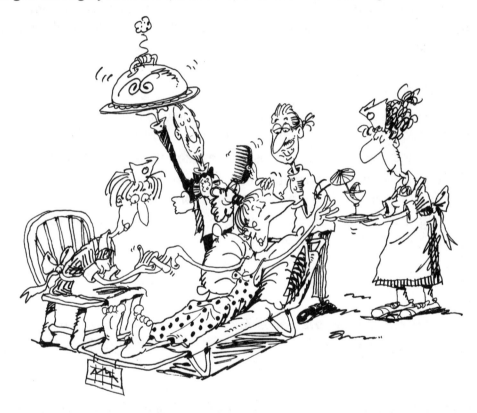

As you breathe in, say to yourself "Cool in," and as you breathe out, say "Warm out." This will distract you from anxious thoughts and also prepare your body to relax. Then continue your slow and steady breathing and as you breathe out let a part of you relax. Start at your toes, then your feet, your legs, your pelvis, then your abdomen and so on, up to the top of your head. Remember your arms and fingers - when you are really relaxing you may feel your finger tips tingle. Relaxation can be assisted with relaxation tapes.* Ask the nurses or physiotherapists if they have any of these tapes.

*The Gawler Foundation for tapes, CDs and courses. Phone Australia 03 5967 1730

TLC - Nature

Nature tops the list of potent tranquillisers and stress reducers. The mere sound of moving water has been shown to lower blood pressure.

Patch Adams

Patch Adams also adds 'art' and 'imagination' to nature as fundamentals of health, influencing the healing for both carer and patient. Yet this has been a largely neglected area in hospital design with gardens often giving way to high-rise buildings and car parks.

A few tips for staying in touch with nature:

- If you can get a room with a view, do! A view of the outside world reminds you of your connection with life, outside the hospital.
- If your hospital has a garden, ask to be taken there by staff or your visitors.
- If you can leave the hospital, even for a short while, visit a local botanic garden or seaside. It will be worth the effort.
- Ask the staff if your visitors can bring in pot plants so you can watch a living thing and wonder at its beauty.

OTHER COMFORTS - Water

We put bubble bath in the baths for our patients. I don't know why it took so long for us to think of it - the patients love it!

Nurse.

A bath, bubble bath, shower or even a simple hand wash from a bowl at the bedside (especially after using a bedpan, or before eating or sleeping) can be a refreshing experience. Sometimes you will have to ask for these things.

Handy Hint: *disposable towelettes are also useful.*

Noise Reduction

Listening to music on a personal cassette player with ear phones can block out noise, or use ear plugs. If you can, ask for your bed to be relocated to a less noisy area.

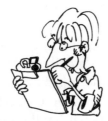

NOTES FOR STAFF

The most frequent cause for complaint by hospital patients is noise: trolleys, voices, phones, and doors banging. People who are sick are very sensitive to noise. (Try sitting on a bed some time and just listen to the amount of noise in your area!) Some hospitals have signs to remind staff and visitors to keep noise to a minimum.

Bedding

Uncomfortable bedding can be transformed to joyous comfort by bringing your own pillow from home. We also suggest a medical sheepskin* which will reduce pressure and discomfort from hard beds and mattresses covered in plastic. A sheepskin for the feet is a great idea if you are in bed for some time. Sheepskins have a natural airing facility and do not make you perspire or feel hot. Some are also urine resistant.

Also consider taking in your own doona or duvet if allowed, so you can regulate the weight and temperature of the bedclothes.

Positioning

A sheepskin can reduce the need for frequent position changes, but there are times when you will feel uncomfortable and you will need to ask for some help. Nurses know how to position you and support you with pillows so you are more comfortable. Don't hesitate to ask them for assistance.

Muscle Tension/Soreness

In addition to massage, the application of local heat will dilate the blood vessels and increase the oxygen supply to an area, thus reducing pain. Local heat is most easily applied with a hot water bottle or a wheat bag (heated in the microwave). Both should be covered and not too hot.

*Fleececraft have excellent medical sheepskins of various sizes and qualities. Mail order. Phone Australia 03 9596 6277

Injection Comfort

If you are to have an injection into your buttock, wriggle your toes and it will relax the muscle. You could also take a deep breath and ask the nurse to give the injection as you breathe out. Make sure the injection sites are alternated from one side of your body to the other. If you have an intravenous cannula (a small tube inserted into your vein), try to have it placed in the hand or arm opposite to the one you use the most. This can be a painful procedure, so ask a nurse to hold your other hand, then take a deep breath - and don't watch! Say to yourself, "I can handle this - all is well."

Oral Comfort

Keep your lips from drying out by using a lip balm or ask the nurses for some lanolin. (If you are allergic to lanolin, try petroleum jelly.)
- A mouthwash improves oral hygiene and can make you feel more like eating.
- Ice chips to suck are sometimes allowed, even if your food and fluids are restricted.

Bedpan Comfort

There is not a great deal you can do about this, but you can put a dressing pad on each side of the pan for comfort.
- If you have a bony spine, try a pad there as well.
- Ask for a pillow for each elbow so you have better balance.

Privacy

- Hospital gowns cause stress through embarrassment! If you have to wear one, ask for two so you can put one on the front and another on the back.
- If you feel upset or you are crying, ask for the screen to be drawn around your bed or the door of your room to be closed.

Constipation Relief

In hospital, a lack of exercise can cause constipation, as can some drugs, especially pain killers (usually containing codeine). Eating fresh fruit and vegetables and drinking plenty of water will reduce the risk of constipation.

You must let the nurses know if you have not had your bowels open in the last 24 hours. Most patients wait too long before speaking up. Nurses have a range of 'aperients' (also known as 'laxatives') with varying degrees of severity which they can give you. Before you take something orally that may cause discomfort as it stimulates the bowel, talk with the nurse about trying a simple suppository.

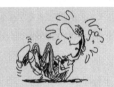

Patient: I'm so constipated, Doctor. I sometimes spend an hour or two in the toilet.
Doctor: Do you take anything?
Patient: Oh, yes: I always take my knitting.

Retrieving!

A simple device for getting things just beyond your reach is a 'Retriever' (claws on a stick) from the occupational therapy department or department store. Your call bell could also be pinned to the sheet so it does not fall off. Many patients also recommend a back-scratcher for that itch you cannot reach!

Pamper

During a series of recent hospital seminars, we had a conversation with a hairdresser. She had a little salon next to the gift shop in the hospital foyer and she also provided hair dressing to patients who were confined to bed. She said the patients love having their hair done and, as much as anything, the light conversation that goes with it. Remember to include life's little pleasures like a hairdo, facial and manicure in your hospital stay. If your hospital does not have these services, the staff may know of a local salon or barber's shop which could send staff into the hospital.

Hospital shop

If you can make it down to the hospital shop, do! They are usually the friendliest places in the hospital. Staffed by caring volunteers who welcome a little chat, and filled with sweet temptations, they provide a welcome relief from the ward environment.

What makes visitors so important is: They buy lollies, fruit and icecream to feed the other visitors who bring the flowers, books and magazines.

Private nurse

Most people agree that hospitals are busy places with overworked staff - especially nurses. One way to overcome this problem is to engage a private nurse to come into the hospital to look after you a shift at a time or for a shorter period. You will need to ask permission from the nurse-in-charge of your ward, and they may recommend a nurses' agency you can contact. Some hospitals supply their own nurses for this purpose (called 'specials'), but only for patients whom they consider to be very sick.

Spiritual

Prayer is powerful aide to healing. Ask if your hospital has a chapel or another quiet place for reflection. Ask to see a representative of your religion, who may visit regularly or on request.

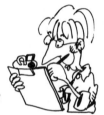

NOTES FOR STAFF

The effect in sickness of beautiful objects, of variety of objects, and especially brilliancy of colour, is hardly at all appreciated. Such cravings are usually called the "fancies" of patients. ... their (so-called) "fancies" are most valuable signs of what is necessary for their recovery. People say the effect is only on the mind. It is no such thing. The effect is on the body too. Little as we know about the way in which we are affected by form, by colour, and light, we do know this, that they have an actual bodily effect.

Florence Nightingale, *Notes on Nursing*, 1859.

Many of the ideas we've included in this chapter are already practised in Palliative care. The question we need to ask is, how we can have more of them in general hospitals.

Old age is not for sissies

– The older person

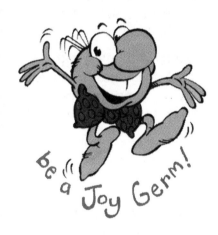

be a Joy Germ!

Show that someone cares

Food for thought

Worried?

Activity

Music, pets, touch and love

Having an operation

Handy hints for visitors

The older person at home

*Since I intend to spend the rest of my life there,
my interest is in tomorrow - and the best thing
about tomorrow is that it comes one day at a time.*

Art Linkletter

IN HIS BOOK *Old Age is not for Sissies*, Art Linkletter shows 'seniors' how to continue having fun, looking good, living well, learning, travelling, taking on new challenges and reaching new goals. Well, if you're to live long enough to do all these things, you had better survive your hospital experience. An experience which, like old age, is not for sissies!

We've included this chapter (the title inspired by Art Linkletter's book) because our years of working in hospitals have convinced us that older people run a greater risk than most other patients of being, to put it gently, 'overlooked'.

Even if you cope well at home, you can quickly become disoriented with the stress of being in hospital. Add to this one or two biological challenges - like poor vision or hearing, or being a little slower on your 'pins' - and you can be disadvantaged as a hospital patient. Not only in getting what you want, but also convincing the staff that you still have all your mental faculties!

Speaking up for yourself can be tough enough when you are younger, but even more difficult and draining when you are older. Some days you just do not have the dash to do it. Our advice is to have someone who is prepared to keep an eye on you and go in to bat for you when it is needed - we'll call them the **'Patient Advocate'**. Don't be afraid to ask your family to do this for you. The ideas in this chapter will show them exactly *how* they can be helpful.

If there is no-one close to whom you can turn for this support, then you need to be prepared to take on the challenge yourself.

*I used to worry about losing my faculties as I
grew older. Then suddenly I realised that if I lost
them, I wouldn't know - I'm much happier now!*

Patient

SHOW THAT SOMEONE CARES - inventing the 'Patient Advocate'

As an Advocate for an elderly patient, you need to convey to the staff on all shifts that you are vitally interested in the progress of 'your' patient. You can do this by visiting or phoning at least every day. Speak to the nurse manager for a full report. Send as many 'Get Well' cards as possible - from family, friends, hostel, nursing home, church, etc.

Let the staff know (it is a good idea to write this down for them):

- The patient's **preferred name** and title.

- The patient's **food preferences** and any **medications** they take.

- Any **assistance** s/he may need with moving, eating, dressing, toileting and hygiene.

- Any **communication challenges** s/he may have with speech, hearing or vision - and what works best to help with these. Bring in spectacles or a hearing aid if it is worn (check battery). You might even put up a sign to alert staff to these challenges.

Handy Hint: *Make sure the call bell is always within the patient's reach.*

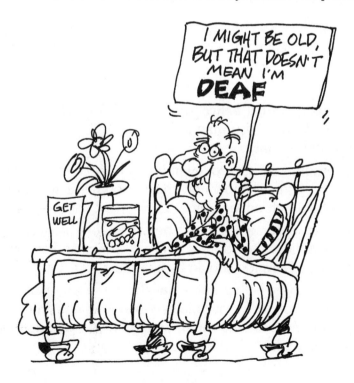

Take in a photo of the patient

A photo of the patient when they were younger is something that always interests staff and makes a big difference to their attitude. It reminds them that the patient was once their age, with a life and personality of their own! Put the photo in a frame on the bedside locker, or tape it to the bedhead.

FOOD FOR THOUGHT (See also Chapter Thirteen)

Nutrition is essential to everyone's recovery, but it is vital for the older person. It cannot be left to chance, because the older person has fewer reserves to draw on and the risk of malnutrition is high.

Robert Morley once quipped that the enemy of old age "...is not death, it is cellophane!" Plastic wrap has taken the place of cellophane as 'the enemy', and many a meal has been on the wrong side of the plastic wrap for a patient to get at it. Let's face it, if the patient cannot *get* to the food, there is not much chance of them *eating* it.

There is a lot that you can do to ensure that *your* patient is properly 'fed and watered' - to their satisfaction as well as yours:

- Discuss food preferences with the hospital dietitian.
- If you can visit at meal times, you can encourage or assist eating.
- Make sure the patient is positioned well for eating and that they can reach the food.
- If there is a long interval between the evening meal and breakfast, then supper is a good idea. You may have to bring this in, or organise for the hospital to deliver a snack.
- Monitor the amount consumed, even if you have to request or start a food chart. This way, you will know how much food has actually been eaten, as opposed to what is left on the tray.
- Dehydration can occur quickly and before anyone notices. Discuss how much fluid the patient should have every 24 hours and encourage him/her to consume this. (This too should be charted.)
- Check with the staff whether fluids have to be in any particular form (eg water only, or no hot drinks, or only low sugar/diabetic drinks, etc). If there are options other than straight water, you can help to top up the supply with more interesting drinks.

- This is also the time to tempt the patient with any favourite foods that you can prepare and bring from home. However, make sure that they are in containers that (a) keep the food fresh, and (b) are easily opened by the patient without assistance!

Studies show that poor nutrition in the aged person will quickly lead to confusion, immobility and a compromised recovery.

Clothes to wear

Easy-to-dress clothing (large openings that fasten) will conserve energy. But keep in mind the importance to the patient of looking good so they will feel better and receive compliments from the staff, visitors and other patients. Label all clothes with the patient's name.

> *You know you're getting old when you stoop to tie your shoelaces and ask yourself, what else can I do while I'm down here?*
>
> George Burns

Constipation

Constipation is a common problem for most people in hospital and particularly the older person. The causes can include inactivity, lack of fibre in food, not enough water to drink and some medications. Encourage your patient to drink lots of water and to have frequent snacks of fresh fruit. Let the nurses know if the patient needs additional help to 'get things moving' (a 'laxative').

> *I wouldn't stay in bed, dear. It's no good lying down, you'll die if you do.*
>
> 90 year-old patient

My doctor's really nice, when I had double pneumonia he only charged me for one.

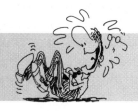

WORRIED ABOUT TREATMENT OR PROGRESS?

Doctors who specialise in treating older people are called *gerontologists*. Not all doctors who look after the aged in hospital are gerontologists. But you can request that your family member or friend be seen by a gerontologist on a public or a private basis. This doctor will assess their condition and response to treatment so far. They will then advise their medical colleagues and let you know how things are going.

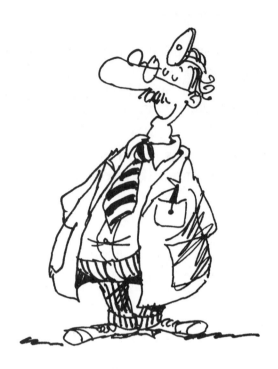

ACTIVITY

- Encourage the patient to do as much as possible without help, especially feeding themselves.
- If they tire as the day goes on, they may be able to manage to feed themselves only early in the day, and appreciate assistance with later meals.
- Discuss planned exercise during the patient's hospital stay with the staff and/or the physiotherapist.
- An outing can serve to reorientate the patient and make them feel better.

MUSIC, PETS, TOUCH AND LOVE...

- **Music** is a great healer and can be quite calming in a strange place, especially if the tunes are the patient's favourites.
- **A patient's pet** from home can restore their spirits and support healing.
- **Human touch** is a powerful healer. Your patient may not be a hugging or touching type, but most people respond well to a gently-held hand, or a stroked arm. It could be that your patient loves having his or her hair stroked, or their back rubbed, or their feet massaged. If your patient responds well to touch, consider organising some **massage** sessions for them.

- If your patient has a strong **faith**, spirituality or religious affiliation, ensure that they either know where the hospital Chapel is, or, if they are not mobile, arrange for a visit from either the pastoral care worker or the hospital Chaplain.

HAVING AN OPERATION

Surgery is a major source of anxiety for the older person. Special care is needed to prepare the patient physically and mentally.

Make sure that the operating theatre staff have contact with you or the patient in advance. At this time you can discuss matters such as previous surgery, how the patient communicates and whether they use any aids to assist movement, hearing or vision. Your visit will always be welcomed by the nurse manager of the operating theatre. You could also ask if you can accompany the person to the operating theatre and stay until the anaesthetic has been given - then wait for the patient in the recovery area.

HANDY HINTS FOR VISITORS:

- **Share the responsibility** for visiting, bringing flowers, sending letters and notes, so it doesn't all fall to the lot of one person.
- Older people sleep less and can be very lonely, so **spread the visits**. A roster works well.
- Try to recall past **happy events** to talk about.
- **Avoid** unloading your worries onto the patient.
- Take in a **'Memory Book'**, an album containing pictures of familiar places and people.
- Take in **magazines and newspapers** that you can browse through together - they are a great source of topics for conversation.
- **Books on tape** are wonderful because the human voice is so calming and comforting. They are available through most public libraries.
- **Avoid appearing to be in a hurry**. The person will sense if you are rushed, tense or annoyed.
- For distant family members consider **recording messages** for them on tape.

Spend as much time as possible with your
'oldie' - you'll never regret those hours.

Daughter

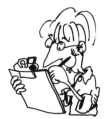

NOTES FOR STAFF

Any disease process or operation has a greater impact on the older patient than it does on those who are younger. Older patients have fewer reserves and their recovery is slower. For this reason they must have the key elements of healing: **nutrition** (including hydration), **rest** and **movement.** Just a couple of days of not eating or drinking properly and they not only lose their reserves, they start developing other problems. Even a simple, untreated, urinary tract infection can cause confusion and disorientation in the elderly. It happens quickly. A record of food and fluid taken is probably more important than any other observation!

NB Make sure the patient's regular and newly prescribed medications are reviewed on admission and before discharge.

Here's some comic relief:

A boy goes to visit his grandmother in a nursing home, and every time he visits he asks her the same question: "Nanna, when are you going to turn into a frog?" His grandmother has no idea what he's talking about, but he keeps on asking. Finally, fed up with all this, Nanna says to him: "Why do you keep asking me when I'm going to turn into a frog?" He replies, "Something dad said. He said 'When Nanna croaks, we're going to Bali.'"

Old age? That's the period of life when you buy
a see-through nightgown and then remember
you don't know anybody who can still see
through one.

Bette Davis

HANDY HINTS FOR THE OLDER PERSON AT HOME

- Use soap-on-a-rope in the shower.
- To prevent dizziness when you are getting up from the lying position, sit for a little while before you stand.
- Any exercise is good, even just rotating ankles and wrists and lifting arms.
- Wear slacks/tracksuits/woollen stockings to protect fragile skin.
- Always wear shoes or slippers.
- See a podiatrist for corns and calluses or problem toe nails. (Especially if the patient has diabetes).
- To inspect the soles of your feet place a mirror on the floor.
- Use thicker pens or pencils for easier grasp.
- Gloves worn in bed at night will relieve arthritic pain.
- Pad the end of a ruler with gauze or similar to dry between your toes.
- Keep your rubbish bin on a luggage trolley to avoid heavy lifting.
- The baby lotion *Nilgard* is good for preventing skin abrasions.
- Dry skin (especially the folds) well and apply deodorant lightly.
- Have your eyes tested once or twice a year.
- Have your local doctor assess all your medications at least *every* three months.
- Don't hesitate to ask your doctor for a referral to a gerontologist to review your condition and management. They can add years to your life! These doctors are available on a public or private basis.
- Use a regulated tablet dosage system from the chemist.
- Have an elevated toilet seat fitted.
- Put rails in the toilet, shower and bath area.
- A shower chair is a useful aide.
- Use a non-slip mat in the shower or bath.
- Use a multi-tap turning device for less effort.
- Pick-up reaching aids are great for retrieval of low-lying or dropped objects around the home.

- A long-handled shoe horn will minimise bending over.
- Wearing gloves for putting on stockings will prevent skin tears.
- Elastic support stockings help prevent leg ulcers or their recurrence.
- Aids are available to help put on stockings, pantihose and socks.
- Continental quilts ('doona' or 'duvet') are lighter than blankets.
- It's easier to get up from a chair with armrests.
- Keep a torch by your bedside (and spare batteries in the drawer).
- You may wake more often in the night as you get older. This is normal. Don't be distressed by it. Just read, have a warm drink of milk then go to sleep when you're ready. (More people die of boredom than of exhaustion!)
- If you get up in the night, put on something warm. It will prevent hypothermia if you fall.
- A commode (portable chair potty) by your bed is always a great idea.
- Keep emergency phone numbers in large print by your phone.
- Personal Alarm Call System which is worn by the person and activated in an emergency. These are available for hire or purchase from suppliers of aides to independent living.
- A cellular phone carried around with you, and at nights a telephone beside your bed, are useful.
- An umpire's whistle around your neck can attract help when needed (provided you tell people about it). Same goes for a personal defence alarm kept in your pocket.
- Grow your vegies and flowers in pots or raised garden beds to minimise bending.
- Velcro tape on clothes and shoes are easier to use than zips and buttons.
- Remember to eat fresh fruit regulary for hydration, nutrients and fibre.
- See the Occupational Therapist for more information on aides for daily living.

My uncle Pat, reads the death column every morning in the paper.
And he can't understand how people always die in alphabetical order.

Hal Roach

Chapter 12

Who cares?
– Caring for the carer

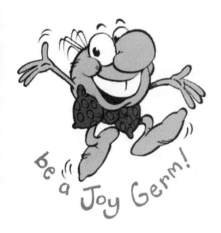

be a Joy Germ!

My elderly mother was fretting in hospital so they sent her home to recuperate. The district nurses helped during the day to bathe my mother, but apart from that it was just me and a 24-hour job. At first I was the one fretting about being able to care for her properly. I got over that in the first weeks, mainly because I was too tired to fret anymore. I let the house go and I let my health go. I was caring for my mother day and night and didn't get time to myself nor enough sleep. The asthma born during that stressful time still plagues me four years later.

Carer

CARING FOR PEOPLE can be rewarding, but it is also demanding and difficult work. In the process, the carer often neglects their own health, thinking 'it can wait', and before long they become stressed, tired and sick.

The message from all carers and their support groups is that **you have to look after yourself so you can keep looking after someone else.** It is easy to get caught up in the routine of the hospital and home and to neglect your own needs. It takes discipline to take time out to meet your own needs.

SPECIFIC IDEAS FOR CARING FOR SOMEONE IN HOSPITAL

- Be specific about what you are doing as a 'carer'. What is your 'job description'? What are you there for that is not done by nursing and other staff?

- Be specific about what you want friends and family to do to help you - and tell them. There are times which may be better spent away from the hospital doing something else for the patient - for example, mowing their lawn.

- On the other hand, if the patient is in hospital for a long time, it is very tiring just getting to the hospital every day. It is a good idea to arrange for family or close friends to share the visiting and to create a roster or timetable. Try saying, "What days will you be in this week...?" Ensure that they understand the time and date as their responsibility!

- Take breaks away from the hospital if you can, or at least away from the unit. Take a walk down the street or into local parks and gardens, so you can experience 'life on the outside'. Even 15 minutes will make a difference.
- Visit the hospital chapel. Prayer - or even quiet time for meditation - always helps.
- Decide what will be left undone at home. Housework can wait, and - if possible - rearrange the remaining chores so other household members can take them on.
- If you find particular visitors are tiring to the patient, ask them not to come in for the moment (or ask the nurses to do it for you) explaining that it is better to spread visitors over a longer period, with less frequent, shorter visits, so as not to tire the patient.
- Try to avoid having the nurses become dependent upon you. Let them know you need some time out.
- When you pass a mirror, give yourself a little wave and a smile. Remind yourself that you're doing your best and that is all you can do.

HOSPITAL AND HOME

Be assertive

For as long as you give the impression you can cope, you will be left to do just that. You have to let people know how you want to be treated, and what you expect them to do.

TIME FOR YOU

What many people fail to realise is the benefit of doing things you love to do. This could include reading, fishing, needlework, walking, watching movies, gardening, talking or just relaxing.

When you are doing what you love to do, it strengthens your immune system (the part of your body that fights disease and keeps you well). Far from being time-wasters, your recreation or hobbies play a vital role in your health and wellness - especially if you are caring for someone else.

Even as a carer, you will still need to make time for these.

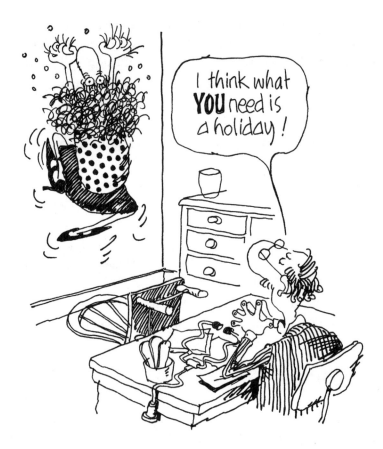

Schedule breaks

The human mind can stand just about anything, so long as it has time out for a little distraction. You cannot 'care' 24 hours a day, seven days a week, without a break. This means organising some relief - ask for help from your family, friends or a respite care service.

I used to think it was selfish to think of myself.
Then one day I heard it called 'enlightened self-
interest' - which means if you can make yourself
happy, you can make others happy.

Carer

LOOK AFTER YOUR HEALTH - Your energy is your greatest asset.

Caring for someone requires lots of energy. When you are in good health you will have more energy and this makes everything you do easier. You need nutritious food, plenty of water, adequate rest and exercise.

- Eat plenty of fresh fruit and vegetables daily.
- High energy foods include complex carbohydrates and these are found in potatoes, rice, pasta, oats and other cereals, wholemeal bread, bananas and corn.
- Cut down on coffee and tea and make sure you have at least six glasses of water every day.
- Getting adequate sleep can be difficult, so it may be necessary to ask a family member to sleep over one night a week. Make sure they can stay long enough to give you a sleep-in the next morning.
- To keep fit, you only need to walk briskly for half an hour each day to feel the physical benefits.
- Just 15 minutes of walking will give you an energy surge for 90 minutes!

Buy yourself some little treats

Treat yourself to a bunch of flowers or a new CD, a massage or facial. Instead of saying you are spending money, think of it as an 'investment' in your well-being, so you can keep on caring.

Remember - a stressed carer is a poor carer.

Who cares?

Loneliness and isolation are some of the hardest parts of being a carer. Help is available! It helps to talk with other people in the same situation. There are Carers' Associations (check with social workers or Health Departments or just look in the phone book) which offer information, training, support and financial advice. Find out what services are available and use them - talk with the district nurses, your doctor, the local Carers' Association, the social worker or welfare worker at your patient's hospital.

Financial security

It is worth investigating any financial assistance schemes for carers run by the government. Carer Support groups usually have contacts for financial or legal problems.

Mental clearance

There will be times when the best way to counter the stress of caring is to indulge in pure fiction. A good movie, video or book can help - *especially if they are funny.* A good idea is to borrow recorded books on tape from your local library, for when you feel too tired to read, but need some distraction.

Acknowledge your feelings

Be prepared for a whole range of feelings, including grief. It is normal and natural to grieve for the loss of something or someone, or some aspect of your relationship that you valued and cared about. You may also feel anger and resentment at having to be on the receiving end of the situation.

*I didn't take him seriously at first. I thought
he was kidding. Then I started to worry and
called an ambulance. Once I realised that
he had had a heart attack I got angry.
How dare he do this to me!*

Wife of patient

There are also positive feelings that come with the privilege of caring for another person.

The highest drug in the world is giving.

Patch Adams

BILL OF RIGHTS & RESPONSIBILITIES FOR CARERS

- Being a carer does not mean you have to sacrifice your whole life for someone else.
- You have a right and a responsibility to take care of your own needs.
- You have a right to be a little bit crazy if it helps.
- You have the right and the responsibility to set limits on how much you are willing to do.
- You have the right to feel, and express all your feelings.
- You have the right to ask others for help.
- You have the right and the responsibility to get professional help when you need it.
- You have the right to do things for yourself.
- You have a right to laugh at any time.
- You have a right to feel lazy.

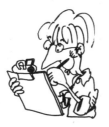

NOTES FOR STAFF

Staff are carers, so the ideas in this chapter apply to you as much as they do to visitors. Too many people balance home and career and neglect their leisure time or private time to do something for themselves. Balancing your life can be a constant challenge. If you can't make your job easier, then perhaps you can make your home life easier by employing a cleaner for a few hours a week. Treasure your friends and make time to play with them, share their interests and express your deepest feelings. Friends are good medicine for carers.

Your Notes

Food for thought
– Your nutrition

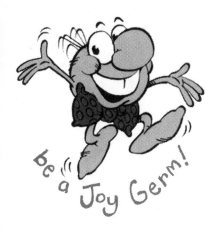

be a Joy Germ!

Food - essential or optional?

Make requests

Choose healthy food

Cut down on tea and coffee

Make eating fun

If you miss a meal

Just add water

Handy hints for hydration

"We all sent out for a pizza the other night, it was great."

Patient

YES, PEOPLE REALLY *are* ordering take-away from their hospital bed. In fact, remember the television commercial that used this theme to promote their pizzas? Why aren't hospitals embarrassed by this? Why do some patients order take-away? Is it because hospital food doesn't taste good? Not enough of it? Served at the wrong time? Or do patients just want a special treat?

Unfortunately the answer is 'Yes' to all of the above. We've worked in enough hospitals to know why most can't get the food right. In short, it is because too many hospitals still consider food to be an optional extra, rather than essential to health and recovery. (Studies show that 50% of long-term hospitalised patients suffer malnutrition!) Some of the food served which is high in fat and protein actually causes stress because it is difficult to digest. There is too little concern with nutrition and too much concern with tray collection.

Yet, food in hospital could be healthy and something to look forward to. In some hospitals you will need to get involved to make this happen.

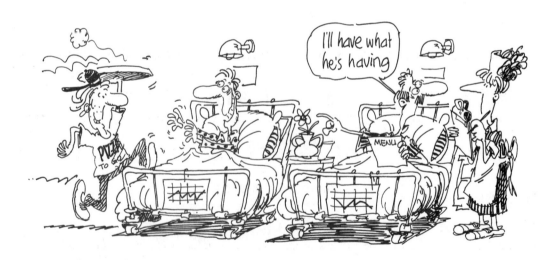

My doctor has more degrees than a thermometer.

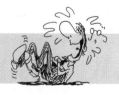

Reaching the food!

You can't eat the food if you can't reach it! If you can't manage to eat your food because you have an intravenous drip in your arm or the tray is too far away - press your buzzer! (Do the same for any other patient you see in this predicament.)

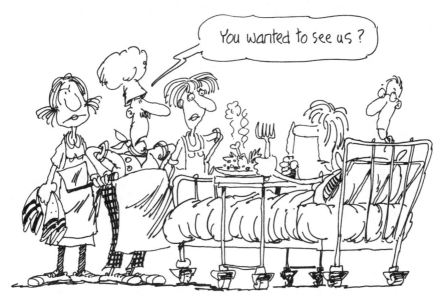

MAKE REQUESTS

- **Ask to speak personally to the dietitian.** These people know the most about the best food to eat for your condition and they can specify what comes on your tray. (Food service staff often only know menu options.)

- **Use your menu as a guide and add any extras you want** - even if you have to attach a note. Even though you may have filled out your menu card the day before, you have a right to change your mind on the day the meal is served.

CHOOSE HEALTHY FOOD

When you are sick, **avoid fried food**.* Choose low fat food, some protein (especially soy products) and a lot of what are called complex carbohydrates. Complex carbohydrates include potatoes, corn, brown rice, wholemeal bread, muesli, beans, lentils, rolled oats, peas and bananas. The body also loves fresh fruit and vegetables.

*Exception: There are some medical conditions in which eating anything, even if it is high in fat, is better than no food at all. There are even conditions in which patients do better on a high fat diet.

CUT DOWN ON TEA AND COFFEE

The trouble with tea and coffee (and cola drinks) is that they contain caffeine and caffeine makes you stressed. It does this by stimulating the secretion of adrenalin - just two cups of coffee is enough to double the amount of adrenalin in your body. The last thing you want when you're sick! The other problem with caffeine is that it is a diuretic which makes you pass extra fluid from your body - another thing you probably don't want if you're sick. So limit tea and coffee to two cups a day and choose alternatives such as herbal tea, water with lemon, diluted fruit juice or decaffeinated tea and coffee.

MAKE EATING FUN!

Get your family and friends involved! Get them to bring in the food that you like if you can't get it in hospital. This can be made appetising by attractive small serves. For example, instead of a big basket of (green) fruit, ask for small pieces of a variety of fruit. (Bring in a big bag of bananas for staff, it will keep their energy levels high.)

Because Sue missed out on a planned dinner party,
we took candles, tablecloth, silverware, glasses and dinner.
The nurses were wonderful - they let us use the common
room and their microwave. We had a ball!

Visitor

Fast food is better than no food.

If you feel like eating hamburgers, ice-cream, chocolate and chips, then eat them. (This is the thinking behind the establishment of McDonald's in children's hospitals.)

"I got my wife to bring in the tomato sauce.
After that I was O.K."

Patient

My doctor told me I'm in good shape for a man of 60.
Too bad I'm only 49.

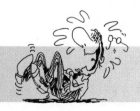

'Grazing' works

When you are sick eating small amounts often seems to work better than the traditional three meals a day. Hold back some prepackaged food from your meal trays and add to it later so you can do this. Remember to have something to eat between the last meal, usually 6pm, and the next one which is 7am or 8am. Find out if the nurses have a toaster in the ward. If they do, all you need is some good bread. (Give them some too, they'll love it.)

IF YOU MISS A MEAL

If you miss a meal because of a procedure, pain or because you were asleep, ask for one to be sent from the kitchen. Don't wait for the next meal time. Sometimes a period of fasting (nothing to eat or drink) can continue indefinately because a test or procedure is postponed. Be aware of this and let someone know. If the food is cold, and shouldn't be, ask for it to be reheated.

Supplementary vitamins

Supplementary vitamins are generally considered to be useful when you are sick. Vitamin C in particular is useful in boosting the immune system and promoting healing. It is often used most effectively when taken in a general multivitamin so other nutrients that may be needed are included.

Avoid choking

Sit up while eating and chew your food well before you swallow it.

For children

Your child's nutrition will not suffer if they don't eat for a few days. If your child's illness is short-term, concentrate on plenty of nutritious fluids and worry less about food. If after two or three days your child is still not eating, make sure the staff know about it. Ask to speak with the dietitian.

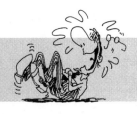

To ensure cleanliness in the hospital, the food you eat is untouched by human hands. But you'll detect a slight flavour of rubber.

JUST ADD WATER

*My 80-year-old aunt had heart surgery recently.
She had a few complications, but was eventually well
enough to come home. After a week or so, she
complained of feeling faint, dizzy and lethargic.
When I asked her how much water she was drinking
and how often she was going to the toilet, the answer
was 'Not much of either.' She took my advice and
started drinking water and her improvement was
remarkable. In her words, 'I feel like a new woman.'
So there you have it - just add water!*

Patricia

We wish this was an isolated incident, but we fear it is not. It is easy to become dehydrated whether at home or in hospital. Dehydration slows healing and can cause complications. Hospitals are usually warm places and the airconditioning causes you to lose water through your skin, even though you are not aware of it. If you drink tea, coffee or cola drinks, you are consuming a drug called 'caffeine', which acts as a diuretic (removes water from the body). The change in your routine which comes with hospitalisation may also mean that you drink less than you would at home.

Why do you need water for health and healing?

Your body is comprised of around 60 per cent water, which is needed for all bodily functions - absorbing oxygen, digesting food, cooling the body, muscle contraction, lubricating the eyes and for healthy skin. You also need water to eliminate toxins from your body and to prevent constipation. You can go without food much longer than you can go without water.

How much water?

There are some medical conditions in which water intake is restricted, so find out if you have one of these. If you do not, you should aim to have six to eight glasses in every 24 hours.

HANDY HINTS FOR HYDRATION

- Ask your visitors to bring in bottles of spring water. Small bottles are easier to handle than large ones or the bulk containers. (In the interests of economy, your most regular visitors could keep a bulk container at home and re-fill your small bottles between visits.)
- If you are dehydrated (because of vomiting or diarrhoea, or simply through not drinking), then sparkling mineral water is more quickly absorbed. However, choose one with no more than 40 mg sodium per litre.
- To add flavour to water, squeeze a few drops of lemon juice or add some mint leaves or a splash of soft drink.
- Avoid sugar-rich soft drinks and undiluted fruit juices.
- As it is easier to drink water on an empty stomach, try to drink some water before your meals.
- Eat fresh fruit and vegetables which are water-rich, especially melon, grapes, citrus, tomatoes, etc.
- Drink herbal or low-caffeine/low-tannin teas instead of 'normal' tea and coffee.

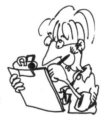

NOTES FOR STAFF

If every patient started requesting special food, some staff may fear that there would be no time to collect the trays. Keep in mind that the aim of a food service is to meet the nutritional needs of patients 24 hours a day - not just delivering three meals a day. Speaking of which, whose responsibility is it to make sure the food reaches the patient and to check what has been eaten?

Just as too many patients are running on empty, so too are staff. Lasting energy foods are the carbohydrates, especially nature's little stress buster, the banana. Ask hospital management to supply bowls of fresh fruit, especially bananas, to your unit for patients and staff. In the scheme of hospital costs, it's hardly an issue.

Your Notes

Laughter medicine
– Shake well

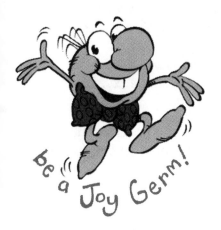

be a Joy Germ!

Laughter - the ultimate stress buster

The benefits of laughter medicine

"Stop laughing, this is a hospital!"

Laughter clinics, fun rooms and silly hospitals

Sense of humour - don't leave home without it

Humorobics - exercising your sense of humour

My friend, Ann, was in a private hospital to have a hysterectomy.
On admission she'd been asked if she wanted a private
physiotherapist to give her some treatment, and she'd agreed.
The first day after surgery the physiotherapist turned up, harassed
and harried and with no bedside manner. The physio must have
been running late, because Ann was still attached to the drip and
the drip stand, and the physio dragged her out of bed, grasped the
drip stand and started to lead her along the corridor.
As they passed the nurses' station, Ann was puffing, pale and
lagging behind as far as her attached arm will allow - while
Super Physio strode out in front with the stand and with little or
no regard for his patient. A nurse looked up in concern and
asked Ann what was going on. Pointing ahead with her free
arm Ann dryly answered: "Just following the Drip!"
If the 'drip' heard the exchange he gave no indication.
Everybody else who heard did - their laughter filled the corridor.

HAVE YOU EVER noticed how much better you feel after a good laugh? It is a total body experience that involves healthy stimulation, then deep relaxation. What could be better to beat stress in hospital?

LAUGHTER - the ultimate stress buster!

A good belly laugh gives you an internal workout. It massages internal organs and improves blood circulation throughout your body, which increases the supply of oxygen and nutrients to tissues. It also improves the function of your immune system (which helps your body to fight disease). For example, the cold virus cannot enter the receptor site of cells when a substance called *norepinephrine* is increased through laughter. (Now there's something to tell your visitors!)

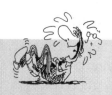

The good part about being in the hospital is getting
breakfast, lunch and dinner in bed. The hard part is
figuring out which is which.

Laughing and chortling help to disrupt your normal breathing pattern so it ventilates the lungs - getting rid of stale air and improving oxygen levels. Laughter leaves your nerves, heart and muscles relaxed. (Including the pelvic floor muscles, which can be a bit of a problem, as they help to support the bladder!)

One of the reasons laughter is so good for you is that when you laugh, you activate the release of biological chemicals called *endorphins* (something else to impress your visitors with) which are the body's natural narcotics - otherwise known as 'pain killers'.

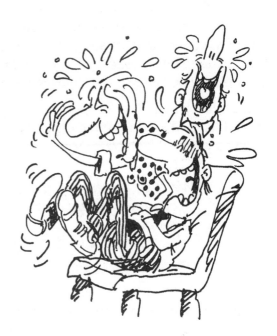

Laughter can relieve pain.

I found comedy helpful. I had friends working in the medical library who sent cartoons to me via the hospital courier.

Patient

"STOP LAUGHING - this is a hospital!"

To get more **laughter medicine** in hospitals, we have to challenge the idea that hospitals have to be serious.

The *work* of hospitals is serious, there is no doubt about that. But that doesn't mean that the *people in them* also need to be serious.

Health care professionals have *serious training* and many have been in strife for having a bit of fun. In consequence, they confuse seriousness with professionalism and put a lid on their sense of humour. This rubs off on patients and visitors - who in turn think *they* have to be serious...

Yet, funny things happen in hospitals. You have strangers coming together to perform intimate tasks. Examinations, tests, treatments and bedpans are just a few of the things that invade privacy and cause embarrassment. Referring to the bedpan as 'The Throne', joking with the staff, and telling stories are common examples of humour that relieves tension.

We believe there is enormous potential for more humour! Deep down the staff *know* this, and so do the patients. What needs to happen is to get it out in the open so we can all enjoy it more.

> *We tried to keep our cardiac unit a little light-hearted*
> *by providing spotty pyjamas for patients to wear.*
> *They loved them - probably more because it reminded*
> *them not to take themselves too seriously.*
>
> Nurse

LAUGHTER CLINICS, FUN ROOMS AND SILLY HOSPITALS

Many health care professionals have recognised the value of laughter and have brought it into hospitals. The first hospital 'fun room' in Australia was established in Maruya Hospital in New South Wales, and Lower Hutt Hospital in New Zealand opened the first 'laughter clinic'. Fun rooms and laughter clinics have a wide range of humour resources - funny videos, joke books, cartoon collections, games, comedy on CD and tape, music, and dress-up bins. Some put on entertainment for patients (and staff!) by way of magicians, comedians and drama groups.

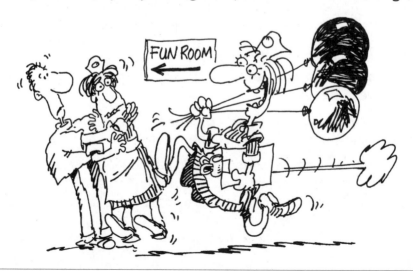

The first 'silly' hospital known as the *Gesundheit Institute*, in West Virginia in the United States, was conceived by Dr Patch Adams. Working all his life for patient-centred health care (and world peace), Patch Adams criticises hospitals for their "sombre atmosphere" and their goal to "fight suffering with suffering." Through the Gesundheit Institute, Dr Adams provides an alternative.

He uses the word 'silly' as it originally meant - good, happy, blessed, fortunate, kind and cheerful. His 'silly' hospital has the healing arts working together - traditional medicine with performing art, crafts, nature, agriculture, recreation, friendship and fun. It is also an eco-village.

Seriousness has no healing qualities at all.

Patch Adams

Let's have what the kids are having!

Children's hospitals tend to be more 'humanised' than adult hospitals. They have more colour, activities, fun, and clowns to visit the patients. We have spoken with enough patients and staff in adult hospitals to know that they want what the kids are having! Send in the clowns!

A sense of humour - don't leave home without it!

Everyone has a sense of humour - it is just that some people have more of it than others. It is clear that in our story of 'Ann following the Drip', Ann has a strong sense of humour. The story also demonstrates that everyone has their own sense of humour or what they find funny. For example, we doubt many physiotherapists will think that story is entertaining! And they would have stories, you, as a patient would not find amusing at all. Have you ever been at the cinema and you're the only person who thinks a line is funny? Then everyone looks at you when the lights come on!

I work in a nursing home as an activities therapist. Just for fun I put knitted teapot cosies on my head. My colleagues accept this, but for some reason they get upset when I put the toilet roll covers on my head!

Allied Health worker

Humour gives us heart. Humour gives us hope.
Humour is a lamp that dispels the shadows
cast by illness.

Robert Holden

It is easy to lose perspective when you are in hospital and sick. You may start thinking that your problem, disease or pain is at the centre of the universe with the whole world revolving around it. That no-one else could possibly feel as bad as you do.

A sense of humour restores perspective so that you can see your problems in relation to the rest of the world. A sense of humour helps you to separate *who you are* from the *problem you're having*. It enables you to take your situation seriously, but not yourself. It doesn't mean laughing it off, but the positive feelings that come from humour will put you in a better position to handle what life hands you.

In a tough situation, instead of saying "I'll look back on this and laugh," (why wait?) ask yourself, "What's funny about this?" If you can't think of anything, ask yourself "What *could* be funny about this?"

I married my husband for his sense of humour.
When the passion fades, you still get a giggle!

Wife

HUMOROBICS - Exercising your sense of humour

If you don't exercise your muscles, they lose tone and waste away. The same thing happens with your sense of humour - you have to use it or lose it! The good news is that you don't have to be naturally funny to boost your sense of humour, nor do you have to be able to tell a joke.

In God we trust and laugh we must.

Sr. Angelica Menta

Comic Relief

A woman was asked, "What made you marry him?" She said, "Opposites attract. I was pregnant and he wasn't."

A man exclaimed, "I'm so proud of myself, I've just finished a jigsaw puzzle." He went on to say, "The reason I'm so proud of myself is because it only took me two weeks, and on the box it said two to four years."

A woman came home from work one day and said to her husband, "I've got good news and bad news about the new car. Which would you like first?" He said, "You'd better give me the good news." She said, "The airbags work."

What tickles your funny bone?

Think about the type of humour you prefer. The range includes puns, slapstick, verbal humour, topical humour, props, gimmicks and things that are not meant to be funny. Once you know your preference, try to find more of it.

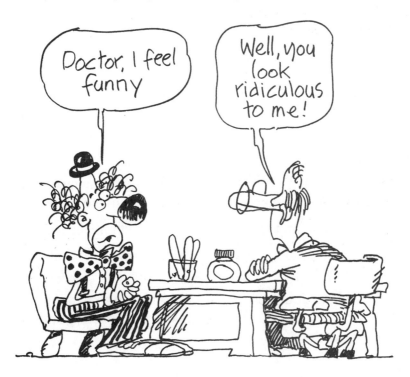

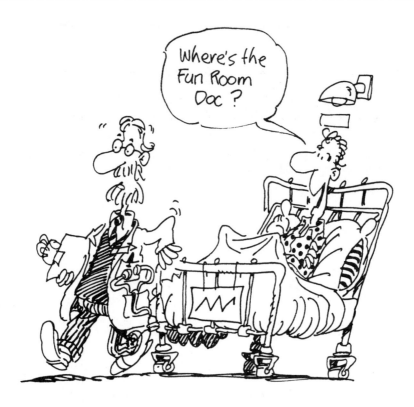

Here's what you can do

- Watch uplifting and funny videos: *The Castle, Liar Liar, Patch Adams, Groundhog Day, There's Something About Mary, Dumb and Dumber, Strictly Ballroom, A Fish Called Wanda, Priscilla: Queen of the Desert, Mr Bean, Naked Gun (all three), Sister Act 1 & 2, Muriel's Wedding, Nuns on the Run, Outrageous Fortune.* Or try old films featuring *Laurel & Hardy, The Three Stooges* and the *Marx Brothers.*

- Ask where the Fun Room is in your hospital!

- In privacy, hold up a mirror and practise making funny faces. When you find the ones that make *you* laugh, then use these to make *other people* laugh.

- Comedy is available on tape and CD - check with music stores and libraries.

- Set up a Fun Club amongst patients, visitors and staff. Call it *'Act Your Shoe Size, Not Your Age'.*

- Get some help from your visitors: ask them to bring something funny with them every visit. Books of jokes, cartoons, novelties, silly hats, puppets, gadgets and games, just for starters.

After my eye operation, my friend made me a pirate's eye patch to wear in hospital. I enjoyed hearing the nurses giggle at it.

Patient

- Brighten your room or bed area with mobiles, funny photos and get well cards. Put up an amusing poster and change it often.

- Find staff members who have a sense of humour and ask them to tell you a joke or funny story.

- Read joke books - mark the good ones and share them around.

- Ask the staff if you can set up a 'Humour Board' in your unit (or put one above your bed) and invite people to put up cartoons and jokes.

- Read the list of fun things to do in 'Notes For Staff' and encourage your team to take risks and have some fun.

Comic Relief

The staff of an inner-city community health centre swear this is true. A very old lady came to the counter. She'd heard of its needle exchange service - what was it? " You bring in your used needles and we replace them," she was told. "What, knitting needles?" "Ah, no," she was gently told.

Column 8: Sydney Morning Herald.

NEWSPAPER HEADLINES:
New study of obesity looks for larger test group.
Red tape holds up bridge.
Police begin campaign to run down jaywalkers.
Plane too close to ground, crash probe told.

REAL SICK NOTES RECEIVED BY TEACHERS:
'Mary could not go to school because she was bothered by very close veins.'
'Please excuse James from PE. He has loose vowels.'
'My son has been told by his doctor not to take PE. Please execute him.'
'Please excuse John for being. It was his father's fault.'

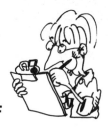

NOTES FOR STAFF

Just as laughter is a great stress buster for patients, so it is for you.

Join in the world-wide revolution to bring laughter, fun and joy into health care. You don't have to wait for everyone else, just do what you can where you are. When you start having more fun on duty, you'll find it will overflow to the patients.

Here are some ideas that we've seen work in many hospitals:

- Dress-up days for staff and patients - everyone has to wear a certain colour, or follow a theme for the day.
- Wacky hat day.
- Celebrations of special days - Christmas in July, Easter, St Valentine's Day, etc.
- Access humour on the Internet (and visit our web site, **www.chy.com.au**).
- Footy picks.
- Start a Humour Board in your unit, in the lifts or cafeteria.
- Parties - any excuse.
- Jokes on meal trays.
- Bring in comedians and clowns to entertain the patients and staff.
- Give special awards for patients and staff who make the effort to lighten the atmosphere.
- Go to comedy clubs and shows together.
- Start meetings with a cartoon at each place or a joke round.
- Send cartoons, chocolate frogs and fish to staff in other departments.
- Do some volunteer clowning or performing - it's fun to play around.
- Read: Robert Holden, who established a National Health Service Laughter Clinic in the United Kingdom and also wrote an excellent book: 'Laughter: the best medicine', published by Thorsons.

I was working in Accident and Emergency and we had a new admission to go to one of the wards - right at the time the night staff were due off duty. So with the patient's file I enclosed a chocolate bar with a note, "Sorry, and thank you!" The next thing I got a call from the night nurse who said, "That's the best thing that's happened to me all night!"

Admissions Nurse

Chapter 15

"I don't like to make a fuss."

– Speaking up

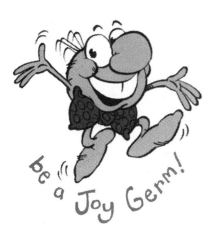

be a Joy Germ!

Ask for what you want

"Doctor, I feel funny."

"No one else has complained."

Handy hints for complaining

The best people to ask for something

What to say

Refusing

Expressing feelings

PICTURE THE SCENE: You needed a bedpan and it took ages for the nurses to answer your buzzer. You waited for it to arrive. You've used it, and now you're sitting on it. Not only are you sitting on it, you're stuck to it! Now, if you've ever been stuck on a bedpan, you'll know the risk involved in self-removal. (It's a delicate balancing act that requires two people, at least one of whom should have some experience in this exercise.) You're going to need a nurse.

You wonder if the one who brought the pan will remember to call back to collect it. Or should you press your buzzer? You know the nurses are busy and probably won't appreciate another buzzer to answer. You sit there feeling stressed and wondering what to do...

If you can sit on one of those bedpans, you should be in Wirth's Circus!

Patient

Or, a more serious example:

The pain was across my chest and down my left arm. I thought it would go away so I waited. I didn't want to make a fool of myself.

Patient having a heart attack

So many people don't speak up because they don't want to 'make a fuss' - they'd 'rather die', and sometimes they do! Let's look at what 'making a fuss' means: *It is getting the attention of professional people who are in a better position than you to decide the seriousness of your condition.* There are only two outcomes when you do this. The first is that you need and get some immediate treatment, and the second is that there is nothing wrong. Either way - you win!

ASK FOR WHAT YOU WANT

It is a fact of life that you get most things you ask for. Yet most people do not ask for what they want in case they will be told 'No'. For many people, the word 'No' makes them feel rejected. However, another way to look at this is to see 'No' as a rejection of your *request*, not of *you*.

"DOCTOR, I FEEL FUNNY."

*I feel funny all the time, but they can't work out
what's wrong with me. So I just get on with my life.*

Former patient

Feeling funny is not always a laughing matter. Nothing gets the attention of a doctor or nurse faster than hearing the words, ***"Doctor, I feel funny."*** It can mean anything from a haemorrhage to a heart attack to a missed meal! So if you feel funny, let someone know.

Also let the nurses know if you are experiencing:

- breathlessness   • feeling sick   • itching/rash
- sweating   • dizziness   • urinary or bowel problems
- tingling   • any discharge   • pain
- anything that you feel is not quite right.

Let someone else decide if your concern is serious or not. Doctors would rather be called to a false alarm than deal with an emergency because you didn't speak up.

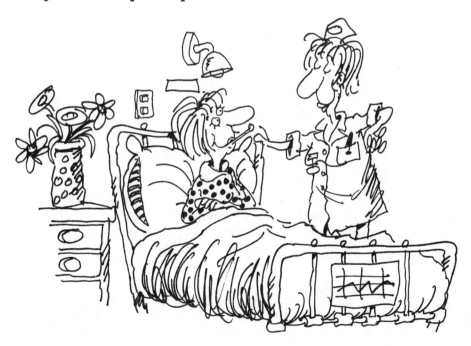

"NO-ONE ELSE HAS COMPLAINED."

Studies show that 96% of unhappy people never complain! That will give you an idea of how reluctant people are to speak up when service falls short of their expectations. Even more so in hospital when, as a patient, you are so grateful to the staff for having saved your life. Add to this the actual or imagined risk of being disapproved of by staff, who have the patient's future in their hands, and you can understand why patients are reluctant to speak up!

The good news is that most hospitals today *are* interested in hearing from dissatisfied patients and have 'customer service' initiatives to deal with complaints. Staff would much rather you speak up so they can be given a chance to solve the problem.

HANDY HINTS FOR COMPLAINING

- Talk only to the people who can help you.
- Speak calmly.
- Say how you feel.
- Let people know what you would like to have happen.
- Say "Thank you" when the problem is fixed.

THE BEST PEOPLE TO ASK FOR SOMETHING

- A friendly staff member - these people often have limited authority but they are prepared to break the rules when they need to.
- The person in charge of the shift.
- The person to whom this person reports - usually a supervisor (day, evening and night) - who covers your area and others.
- The person in charge of the service with which you have a problem (the nurses can tell you who this is).
- The Director of Nursing or the Hospital Manager. These people are rarely consulted by patients but love to get involved. So, find out their name, then say to the nurse manager "I would like to see Mr Wannahelp. Would you mind arranging that for me please?"

I always thought talk was cheap until I started talking to a psychiatrist...

WHAT TO SAY

Often we don't make requests because we're just not sure of the words to use. So be *clear* about what you want. Here are a few examples:

- "Anne, I'd like to talk to you about something that's on my mind. Could you see me when you have few minutes to spare?"
- "Nurse, would you mind removing my husband's bedpan please, he's finished with it. Thank you." (Smile!)
- "Miss Jones, could I have something for my pain, please?"
- "Would it be possible to have a room on my own, please?"
- "Nurse I don't feel well. It's hard to explain, but I know I need to see the doctor as soon as possible." (The nurse may say he's very busy.) "Yes, I'm sure he is busy and I'd appreciate you letting him know I need to see him."
- "Nurse, I'm not getting along with the other patients in this room. May I be moved, please?"
- "I know I've had a pain killer already but it isn't controlling my pain. Could I have something different, please?"
- "Nurse, what are these tablets for?"

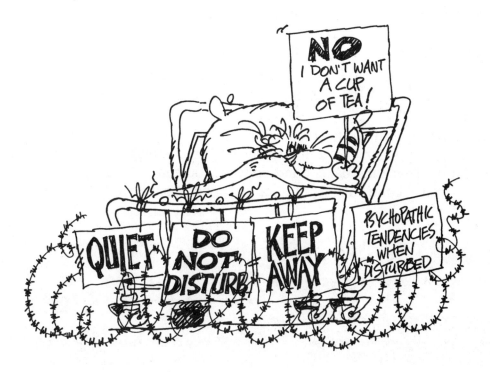

REFUSING

If you are not happy about your treatment or something that the staff expect you to do, you have a right to refuse. This is how you might say it:

- "I know the doctor has prescribed those tablets nurse, but I'm not happy taking them."
- "I know students must learn, but I don't feel up to seeing them today."

EXPRESSING FEELINGS

People cannot read your mind. If you feel unhappy about a situation you need to say so. For example:

- "My doctor led me to believe I would have my own room. I feel disappointed that I've got to share."
- "When I'm served a meal I can't eat, I feel annoyed. Please could I have a salad instead."
- "When you take the time to explain what's happening, I feel reassured. Thank you."

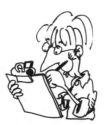

NOTES TO STAFF

The important thing to remember about complaints is to take them *professionally*, not *personally*. If you have ever complained you'll know how stressful it is. Thank the patient and do what you can to fix the problem. Then, take steps to make the patient or visitor feel good about having spoken up.

Notes written by student nurses:

"Mrs Jones ate a little jelly; vomited a trifle."

"Betty Brown has been vomiting frequently all day. I understand she is expecting her sister up this evening."

"Mrs Smith doing well, but baby not so good. Taking breast badly. Poor sucker!"

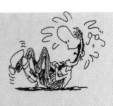

Chapter 16

Tell me more 16

– Getting information

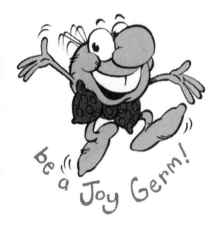

be a Joy Germ!

I forgot to ask...

Getting the doctor's attention

Getting information

Questions to ask

Patients' Bill of Rights

*I couldn't get the information I needed, so I used
my bedside phone to call the hospital and
pretend I was my father. That way I got more
information about me ('the son') than me ('the
patient') than I had in days!*

Patient

THIS STORY MAY sound extreme, but getting information in hospital sometimes requires extreme measures. It will certainly mean that you must get involved in asking questions and persevering until you get the answers.

People worry that too many questions about their treatment will be misinterpreted by the staff as not having confidence in them, or that it will lead to indifferent care. This is not the case.

Your reward will be less stress and more control. You will also reduce some of the potential risks of being in hospital, including mistakes, misdiagnoses, medication errors, and unnecessary tests.

"I FORGOT TO ASK THE DOCTOR..."

Sometimes what happens is that you think of all the questions you want to ask the doctor, but the minute the doctor arrives, often with a gaggle of students and nursing staff, your mind goes blank. As soon as the doctor leaves, all the questions come back to you.

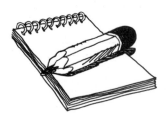

Keep a notebook in your locker and, as you think of each question, write it down. When the doctor arrives, you have all of your questions, thoughts and ideas in front of you and they can be ticked off as the doctor responds.

A hypochondriac is a non-golfer who joins a country club because it's the only place he can find a doctor on Wednesday afternoons.

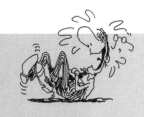

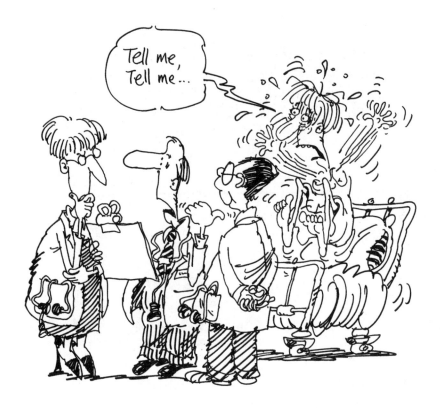

Words to use

Sometimes knowing what words to use can help you to ask questions. Here are some examples:

- "Doctor, I don't understand what's wrong with me. I know you say you're not sure yet, but I'd like to know what you *think* is the problem."
- "Could you please explain to me what that means?"
- "I think I'll do better with this procedure if you explain what's involved before you start."
- "Nurse, I'd like to speak with a nurse from the operating theatre before my operation. Could you arrange that please?"

GETTING THE DOCTOR'S ATTENTION

Sometimes the best way to get information is to make an appointment with the doctor or specialist (in the hospital or at their practice), especially if you are the carer. "Doctor, I wonder if I could make an appointment with you please to discuss my husband's condition?"

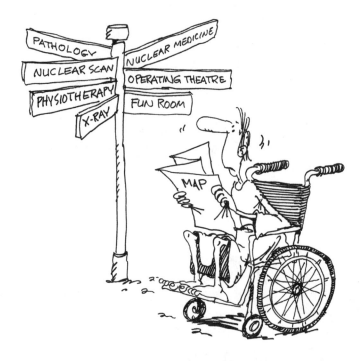

GETTING INFORMATION ABOUT PROCEDURES
(including your operation)

Where to look for information:

There is a wealth of information available - you just have to be prepared to hunt it out! Try these for starters:

- Your doctor or surgeon. If they are rushed, make another appointment just to have explanations.
- Health care professionals including natural therapists.
- Support and educational associations such as the National Heart Foundation.
- Support groups set up by patients and their families.
- Hospital resources - videos, information booklets, texts and articles - especially if the hospital has a patients' library.
- The department in which the procedure is performed - they often have leaflets with an explanation specific to your condition.
- Your local library, which can arrange an inter-library loan from medical libraries.
- The Internet and the World Wide Web - rich sources of information on both the procedure and the locations and activities of common interest groups nationally and internationally.

*Become a student of your disease. As soon as I
started asking the right questions in a way that
showed I knew a bit, doctors shifted from being
paternalistic to acting like colleagues.*

Norman Cousins

General information about having a test or X-ray

- If you are having pain relief medication, ask for some before you leave the ward. (Moving around on an X-ray table can be painful).
- Most people have their best energy reserves in the morning, so ask if you can have your procedure or test then.
- A voluntary consent form many need to be signed for some tests.
- You may be transferred on a trolley or in a wheelchair even though you can walk. (This is a safety precaution.)
- It may not be the same porter who takes you to the department and picks you up.
- Expect a delay after your X-ray or test and before returning to your ward while the porter is phoned and arrives.
- It's a good idea to have a family member with you if the procedure is in another department and is a long one. Departments don't always have the staff to get you what you need.
- You may feel tired after your procedure.
- If you miss a meal, ask for one when you return.

*It's embarrassing having people stare at you when
you're being transported around the hospital.
Having a magazine to look at does help.*

Patient

Creative sign in X-ray: "We'll see you through!"

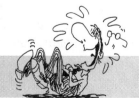

How does your doctor rate as a communicator?

Does your doctor:

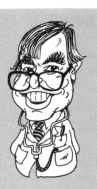

- ask *open questions* which allow you to tell the whole story? (Open questions start with words like *how, what, tell me about, when,* etc.)
- listen without interrupting?
- let you know the reasons for a diagnosis and treatment?
- ask background questions about your history, family, and lifestyle?
- look at you when you are talking, and appear interested?
- use language you can understand?
- encourage you to ask questions?
- admit "I don't know," when appropriate?
- give you choices and take account of your preferences?

If your answers show more 'No' than 'Yes' answers, then your doctor doesn't communicate well. Now you have a choice:

Option 1:   *Find another doctor.*

Option 2:   *Take a deep breath, be calm, and be honest with your doctor. Explain how you feel about their style. Tell him/her that you <u>do</u> have trust and confidence in their medical proficiency, but you are not happy with the lack of openness between you. Show your doctor the above list - and then suggest a 'partnership for healing' which involves the two of you being honest and open with each other, and more willing to share feelings and information.*

They tell you to breathe in then 'Hold it there for three seconds', but don't tell you when the time is up!

Patient

QUESTIONS TO ASK ABOUT YOUR OPERATION

- Where will I wake up? Then where will I go?
- How do most people feel after this type of operation?
- Will I have a blood transfusion?
- Will I have intravenous therapy? (A needle in your arm which slowly feeds fluid into your body to administer medications and to keep you hydrated until you can drink again.) For how long?
- Will I have one or more drains? (A drain is tubing left in the operation site to drain away any discharge.) For how long?
- Will I have a tube in my mouth? For how long?
- Will I have a catheter? For how long?
- How big will the wound be? Will the stitches have to be taken out, or will they dissolve? When?
- Will I be connected to any machine or monitor?
- What pain relief will I have and how will it be administered? (tablets/intramuscular/intravenous infusion.)
- Will there be a scar or scarring?
- Is there anything else I need to know?

What you should know about tests and procedures

- What the test or procedure is for.
- What it involves.
- If you are likely to experience any pain or discomfort.
- Whether the potential advantages of the test outweigh any risks.
- What will happen if you do not have the test or procedure.
- Whether a sedative, local or general anaesthetic or will be used.
- Where it will be performed.
- The cost.
- How long it will take.
- Whether you can go home or back to work afterwards.
- Whether you can drive or use public transport alone, or if you will need assistance to get home.

Access to your file

If, after all this questioning you are *still* not getting answers, then the *Freedom of Information Act* in Australia (*Privacy Act* in New Zealand) gives you the right to access your medical records if you were treated in a public hospital. The hospital requires your request in writing and has the right to review the record before you read it. Such a request usually leads to fast action from the clinical staff, who may then be more motivated to answer your questions!

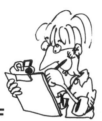

NOTES FOR STAFF

We have seen the patients' libraries at Stanford Medical Centre in the United States. They work very well and there is even one of these in the local shopping centre. At first, the doctors were concerned that patients and their families would be confused by too much information, but they need not have worried. They discovered that *informed patients are easier to communicate with and treat.*

Alternatively, much of the information patients need can be recorded on tape, video or printed in leaflets. They may take time to prepare but they save time in the long run, especially when you have inexperienced staff on duty.

Did they really mean that?

From Doctors' dictating machines:

"Patient states that she was bitten by both legs of a dog."

"The patient had reportedly been doing very well when, after breakfast, she suddenly lost her right arm and was unable to speak."

"The patient has never been pregnant and denies any reason for this."

"On the second day, her knee was better and on the third day, it completely disappeared."

"The patient wears glasses for hearing."

"Patient is a real gas factory."

Internet

PATIENTS' BILL OF RIGHTS

You have the right to...
- physical privacy.
- confidentiality relating to any information you share with staff.
- dignity and respect as a human being.
- a reasonable level of care.
- be in a safe environment.
- have a say in what is to happen to you.
- clear and understandable information.
- ask for a second opinion.
- be alone.
- know the names and positions of people who are involved in your care.
- practise or participate in your chosen religious or spiritual preferences.
- legal rights as a member of society.
- refuse to be examined by students.
- refuse treatment.
- use the information and ideas in this book.

Hospitals have the right to expect that you will...
- share information (from you or your family) to assist your care and treatment.
- speak up if you are concerned about your condition or require additional medication (eg pain relief).
- comply with treatment recommended.
- be responsible for your actions if you refuse treatment.
- be considerate towards other patients and staff.

Try to care for your caregivers, no matter how poorly other health care professionals may have treated you in the past. Try to be relaxed, respectful (not worshipful), and forthright. If a healer acts in a way that bothers you, speak up gently but firmly about your concerns.

Patch Adams

Your Notes

Mum's the word

– Having a baby

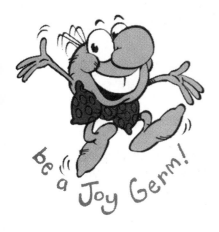

be a Joy Germ!

There was a picture of Mt. Buffalo in the delivery room - it was my focus point. Bad choice! The more I looked at it the more convinced I became that whoever was inside me was about the same size and here was me trying to push it out of an opening the size of a pinhole! At about the halfway mark I decided I'd rather do this another day; I didn't want to play any more. By the second stage, I knew buying a puppy was an option I should have investigated more thoroughly - and that the nurse hovering over me who kept reminding me that 'women do this every day', was in real danger of meeting an early death!

Then he arrived. My baby. And I held him in my arms, and all the stories I'd heard about it being all worthwhile in the end came floating back.

Then the doctor started inserting the stitches...

Mother

MOST ASPECTS OF having a baby are covered in prenatal classes, but no matter how prepared you think you are, there will be times when the whole thing will seem utterly overwhelming. What we've included here are ideas to take the stress out of being in hospital so that having a baby is more enjoyable.

In the last weeks of my pregnancy, I was saturated with books and good advice on childbirth and parenting.

Mother

A sign on the maternity ward door:
PUSH! PUSH! PUSH!

Extract from an essay written by a student nurse:
"A woman who is expecting a baby should always go to her local doctor as soon as she has reason to believe that she may be pregnant. She must realize that her local doctor is always the person mainly responsible for her condition."

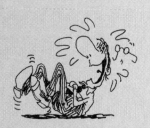

WHAT TO BRING

You'll have a standard list of baby and medical requirements. Add to these:

- A doona or duvet for your comfort and adequate warmth.
- A set of baby clothes, nappies and blanket to bring your baby home in.
- The 'baby capsule' for the car. (Ensure bolts and accessories have been fitted correctly prior to the day of discharge).
- Camera and film.   (Check the batteries too).
- Something light to read during quiet moments and rest periods.
- Bubble bath, soap and body lotion - make use of the bath in the ward and treat yourself to a relaxing bubble bath.
- Comfortable street clothes and flat shoes - you do not have to spend your time in a nightdress and gown. Extra pairs of panties to save washing. (Disposable ones if finances permit).
- Your favourite tea, herbal tea or coffee - add to this something to eat. Most mothers are starving after giving birth!
- Money, including change for phone calls - you'll have plenty to make.
- 'Thank you' notepaper or cards, postage stamps.
- A clock or watch - breast feeding in most hospitals is no longer timed, but it will help to know what time of day it is!
- Hairdryer - useful for drying your perineal area if you have stitches.
- A roll of very soft toilet tissue!
- A sheepskin to sit on, which can later be used at home for the baby.
- Torch and spare batteries.
- Your sense of humour!

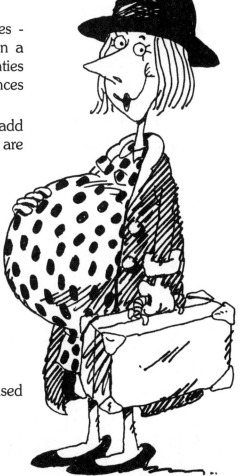

WHAT MOTHERS SAY...

This was the instruction given to me by the midwife running our prenatal class: 'Wear the oldest possible underwear. I don't want to see any silk or anything pretty.'

My advice is to wear dark-coloured lycra - it hides everything!

I was told to leave my modesty at the front door of the hospital and collect it on the way out!

WHY WOMEN HAVE A STRONG SENSE OF HUMOUR

We are convinced that women laugh more often than men. We presume that the reason for this is that our Maker blessed women with the stronger sense of humour because they need it. For example, when a woman is having a pap smear and the doctor says, "Just relax." Or having a mammogram... now there's a machine invented by a man! (We think they should have one for themselves - invented by a woman!)

And now you're giving birth and you're told "Just breathe." (Yet if a man has a headache he wants an ambulance!)

One thing is for sure, you are going to need a sense of humour to give birth.

Having a baby is like being on a hormonal roller-coaster. Add to this the physical and mental impact of actually giving birth (especially for the first time), and it's understandable that you're going to have some unpredictable emotions.

In tough situations, ask yourself "What's funny about this?" Humour restores perspective. So does crying, so if all else fails, have a good cry.

I went to the Birth Centre in the hospital. It was much more relaxed and casual, more like at home.

Mother

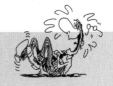

My doctor advised me to give up those intimate dinners for four unless I had three people eating with me...

HOSPITAL MIDWIVES

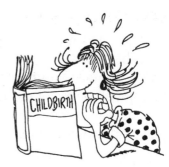

For you, giving birth is one of the most important events in your life. For hospital midwives your delivery, although very special, is just one of many. You will find most of the hospital staff kind and considerate, but some will also tend to take control and give advice. There are times when you want this, especially if it will save your life, but at other times, you may resent it.

Another challenge is the confusion that can arise from midwives' differing views on different shifts. Be prepared by being well-informed: read up on childbirth before you come into hospital. Clarify any conflict of opinions by asking to see the manager of the unit or the clinical nurse consultant for the area.

The best advice I ever had came from a pharmacist who said, 'Listen to advice - but follow your own instinct. Most times whatever the mum feels is right for her baby, usually is. They don't call it maternal instinct for nothing.'

Mother

You know more than you think you do.

Dr Spock

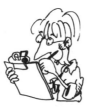

NOTES FOR STAFF

Mothers tell us that one of the most frustrating and confusing aspects of having a baby is conflicting advice from midwives. We have seen some midwifery units which have overcome this problem by implementing clear protocols about breast feeding, debriefing for mothers, post delivery and routine aspects of post natal care. They also provide staff and patient orientation education (especially staff orientation) and comprehensive staff handovers.

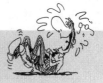

Have you heard about the baby born in the high-tech delivery room? It was cordless.

YOUR OWN MIDWIFE

This is an option you may want to consider. Midwives in private practice are available to assist you throughout your pregnancy and hospitalisation, and when you go home. Your midwife will accompany you to hospital and support you through all stages of labour and delivery. This overcomes the problem of having to cope with different staff on each shift in the hospital. Your own midwife consults and works with the hospital midwives, but s/he is there just to be with you.

Let your obstetrician and hospital staff know ahead of time that you wish to have your own midwife with you (although it is never too late to bring one in).

Some private health funds will pay for private nurses. If they don't, why not suggest to friends and family that they club together to pay some of the private nurse consulting fees? This may be more beneficial than some other gifts.

To contact registered midwives: Telephone the *Australian College of Midwives* or *New Zealand College of Midwives.*

Be prepared but flexible

In addition to completing the pre-admission form, it's a good idea to visit the maternity unit to meet the staff ahead of time. You can discuss how you expect the labour will progress - what things you can do in labour, positions in labour, pain relief, etc. You have to have some idea of what is available before you can say what you want!

I had my baby on all fours on a mat on the floor. I'm sure that if the doctor had arrived in time, he would have insisted I lie on my back on the bed.

Mother

This is a true story told to us by a midwife at a seminar in New Zealand:

I was on an evening shift with a friend. She goes into a patient's room to find a blood test result. The patient - who hasn't delivered - is sitting up in bed and her husband is sitting on the chair next to her. The midwife goes through the patient's file and can't find the test result. Finally, in exasperation, she says "Well, there's been a cock-up here!" She was so embarrassed she couldn't go back into the patient's room for the rest of the shift...

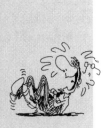

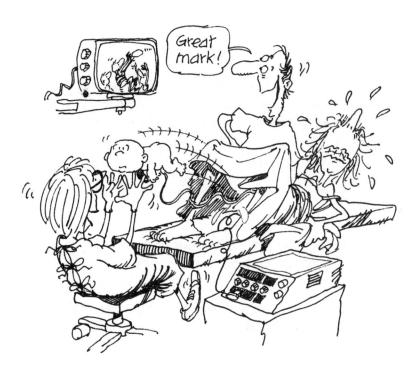

GET YOUR PARTNER OR SUPPORT PERSON INVOLVED

These people can assist in many ways. For example, massaging any aching areas of your body, providing cold face washers, offering regular food and fluids (as permitted), meeting your requests and generally keeping your spirits up! Keep in mind that even the best support person may feel inadequate at times when you are having difficulty conveying your needs between contractions.

If your birthing partner or support person is looking for something useful to do in the last months of your pregnancy (having completed the childbirth preparation and parenting courses!), suggest s/he do some assertion training! These skills can be very useful when speaking up for you, as your advocate, when your reserves are low.

It is usual for your partner or support person to be involved 'hands-on' in the actual birth, but it is still an individual choice. It is acceptable for the person to change their mind at the last minute!

I would have liked a course in nappy changing.
Not only in the technique, but in developing a
constitution for it!

Father

VISITORS

Why is it that when you're in hospital, people come to see you and expect you to entertain them? After each visiting time, I felt like I had just finished a Command Performance. I was exhausted. The visitors toddle off home, happy with their lot - while my 'lot' is screaming her little head off.

Mother

Visitors can be tiring and you may want your privacy to get to know your baby. Let your family and friends know how you feel about visits before you go into hospital, and consider asking some of them to visit you later at home.

(The same applies to flowers, pot plants, cutesy stuffed animals and huge cards - they are much more welcome at home and less likely to be knocked into the soup!)

Rest

The reality of hospitals today (public or private) is that as a mother you will get little rest in hospital. Therefore, you must make plans to get as much rest as possible when you go home.

Needing rest is also a great way to allow people close to you to contribute. Tell them *how* they can help, especially in the first few weeks you are home - perhaps picking up shopping (either with a list or collecting pre-ordered goods from the supermarket); household laundry (not the nappies - that may strain the bonds of friendship too far...); taking you or the baby or the dog to the park or out for a drive; mowing the lawn or weeding the garden to keep it neat for you; a spot of vacuuming or house-cleaning; taking to or picking up your other children from school, or sports practice, or social functions. Good old-fashioned 'babysitting' can be a huge help too.

The telephone

Too many phone calls can delay establishing a routine of events both in hospital and at home. Consider delaying telephone calls to all but close family and friends until after discharge. Ask people to contact your partner or your mother (rather than you), both of whom will be yearning to tell everyone the whole story.

An inexpensive and companionable alternative is a **'telephone tree'**. Before you go into hospital, write all the relevant names and numbers on a piece of paper and then allocate two or three calls per 'branch'. The first person you tell about the birth starts off the 'tree'. This way, lots of people get to talk to each other about your great news, and no one person is burdened with giving out expensive, time-consuming and ultimately very repetitive information about the 'happy event'!

BACK HOME - remember to eat and rest

- Your body needs nutrition at this time, and it is easy to miss a meal because you're feeding the baby. Salads are good because they are nutritious and easy to prepare. Hopefully, you or a friend may have been able to prepare and freeze some meals before the birth. Pop them in the microwave or leave in the fridge overnight to defrost - instant food!
- Complex carbohydrates are 'energy foods' and found in bananas, wholemeal bread, rice, corn, potatoes, oats and potatoes.
- Every baby is different and it can take a while to establish a home routine, so grab whatever rest you can, when you can. There's nothing wrong with occasional cat-naps, even if they're only 10 minutes!

Your Notes

Sheepless nights
– Getting sleep

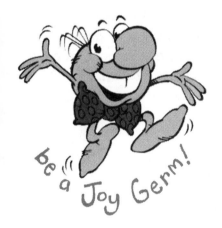

be a Joy Germ!

The importance of sleep

What to bring from home

'Top Ten' ideas for sleep

The ABC method for getting back to sleep

Other ideas

What you need is a full-face crash helmet with tape on the visor to get sleep in hospital.

Sleep-deprived patient

EVEN IN A hospital, which defies all rules of nature, night must fall. There was a time when hospitals did what they could for you, then you were left alone to rest and - hopefully - recover. All that has changed in todays stressful hospital environment. Most of what goes on in a hospital works *against* rest and sleep. Noisy air conditioning, treatments, tests, phones ringing, staff chatting, patients snoring, doors banging, beepers beeping and trolleys squeaking... all that seems to be missing is the screech of cicadas!

The bed itself is designed more for action than rest. It is narrow, high and hard. This is a good thing if you need emergency treatment because it comes into its own as a procedure table! The mattress and pillow covers are usually made of stiff protective plastic which is uncomfortable and crackles everytime you move.

Sleep is vital for recovery and to give you the strength and energy to continue tests and treatment. Not having enough sleep can make you feel irritable, confused, and more sensitive to pain. Sleep deprivation causes stress and weakens your immune system (that system in your body which fights disease and helps healing).

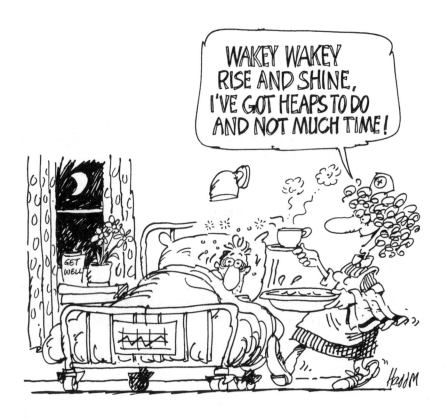

We've seen patients who, in intensive care units were considered to be 'hopeless'. Once transferred out of this hectic environment to a single room in a ward, they caught up on the sleep they couldn't get in the intensive care unit. Many of these patients surprised the doctors by getting well!

Turn your 'action' bed into a 'comfort' bed by bringing in from home:

- A favourite pillow (with favourite pillowslip).
- A sleeping mask and ear plugs (from the chemist).
- Herbal teas.
- Continental quilt (comforter/doona/duvet) if allowed.
- Sheepskin to lie on (if the hospital doesn't have one).

*What I really hated was being woken at 6.00 am
and asked how I slept...*

Patient

HERE ARE OUR TOP 10 IDEAS FOR GETTING SLEEP IN HOSPITAL:

1. Try to get a position away from the nursing utility areas, especially the office and the panroom. Asked to be moved if you're disturbed by other patients or their treatments in the night.

2. If you need pain relief, ask for it approximately half-an-hour before sleep.

3. Prepare for sleep by reading a light novel or magazine, or listening to an audio book or music. This tells the body it is time to sleep. Avoid watching television. Far from being relaxing, it can be very exhausting.

4. Hunger can keep you awake. If you're hungry ask for food which is high in carbohydrate and low in fat and protein. A ripe banana, bread or toast. Chamomile and other herbal teas are better than caffeine drinks such as hot chocolate, tea, coffee and coke.

5. Write a 'Do not disturb' sign and put it on your bed head or pin it to the bedclothes.

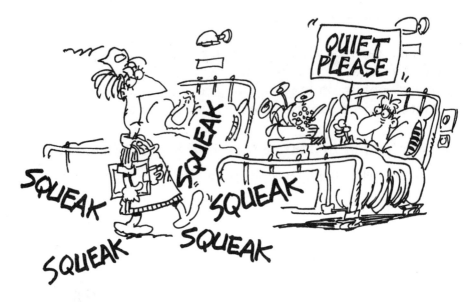

6. Wear a sleeping mask. Not only will this block out the light, it will deter people from talking to you.

7. Try to get up and walk around in the day. Physical tiredness is the number one factor for sleep promotion.

8. Ensure your bed temperature is comfortable. If you're too hot or too cold you'll have trouble sleeping. Ask for extra blankets if you need them.

9. Accept the need for an occasional sleeping tablet.

10. Ask the staff to contact the engineering department to fix noises near you, such as squeaking doors, etc.

Did you hear about the dyslexic, agnostic, insomniac?
He lay awake all night wondering if there really was a Dog...

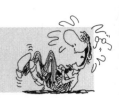

Can't sleep a wink?

If you start worrying about not getting to sleep, it will only make things worse. Once you start worrying, you get stressed. 'Resting' can be just as beneficial as sleep.

THE ABC METHOD OF GETTING TO SLEEP

A for **Awareness:**

Be aware of the thoughts that are keeping you awake.

B for **Breathing:**

Breath deeply and relax your body. If you're in pain, 'breathe into the area' and release the pain as you breathe out.

C for **Change your thoughts:**

Choose new thoughts. "I'm in good hands and I'm going to sleep." Say this to yourself repeatedly. Or try, "I'm very tired and I'd like to be asleep." If the 'worry' thoughts come back, let them go and choose some new, relaxing ones.

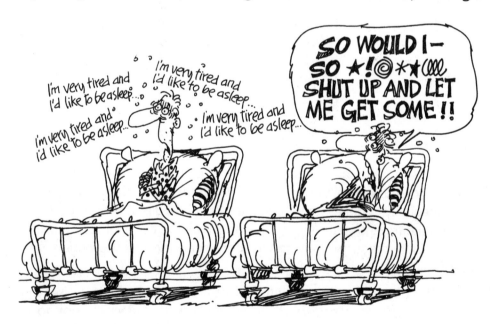

Books on tape

We think these are the best inventions ever for patients in hospital. There are some wonderful titles available and they are easily borrowed from a local library. Just plug into a personal cassette player and enjoy the soothing effect of the human voice and something other than yourself and your condition to think about. Talk back radio can also be soothing.

Ask for a massage

Just a simple shoulder, foot or hand massage will help sometimes.

Try some new thoughts

- **Imagine** you're working on something at home - weeding the garden, fixing your car, cooking, etc.
- **Imagine** someone who is soft and warm and will hold you in their arms all night long.
- **Imagine** you're back at school. Think of particular friends and imagine what they're doing now.
- **Imagine** you're at your favourite holiday spot. Get involved in the things you like to do most - smile, relax and have some fun.

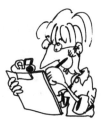

NOTES FOR STAFF

Shift work is stressful, especially working on night shift. We once did a seminar series for night nurses called *A Little Night Relief* in which we declared night nursing a speciality. It takes knowledge and special skills to promote sleep, decide when to initiate treatment and to work without all the hospital resources available in the day. Only when *you* are taken more seriously will the *patient's sleep* be taken seriously.

Noise is the biggest barrier to getting sleep in hospital. *Even noises that don't actually wake patients, can disrupt the normal cycle of sleep.* Look to the little things that you can do to minimise disruptions to sleep: such as putting a towel on top of trolleys; getting wheels and door hinges oiled; keeeping conversation amongst yourselves to a minimum; changing times of observations to 10pm and 8am instead of 12 midnight and 6am.

Bed bugs and bear hugs

– Your child in hospital

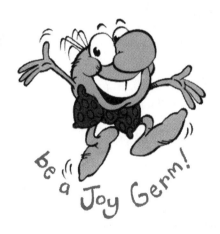

be a Joy Germ!

Things to do before your child is admitted to hospital

What to ask hospital staff

What to pack

When your child is having an operation

Visiting children in hospital

Things to play with

Going home

THERE IS NOTHING very amusing about your child going into hospital. Suddenly your big, brutish seven-year-old looks very tiny in that big hospital bed, and you notice the baby features you thought he was outgrowing are very much in evidence again. And the hugs he's been telling you he's too big for are now a little longer and tighter, and the jokes about bed bugs don't seem as funny when he's in a strange bed. And that's just how *you* feel... Can you imagine how *he* must be feeling?

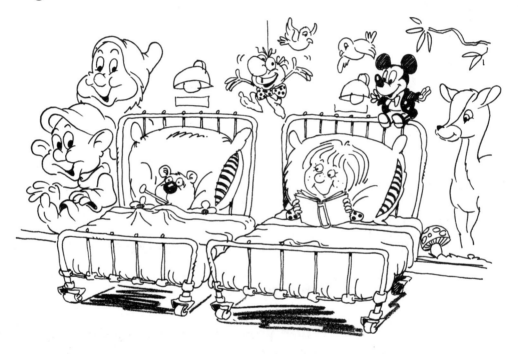

To a child, going into hospital is a potentially traumatic and stressful experience. Just as adults fear the unknown, so do children. The aim of supporting a child in hospital is to reduce the psychological distress associated with this new experience. The more information *they* have, the less distressed they'll be. The more information *you* have, the more you'll be able to help your child.

Remember: *you are the model and the child will follow your lead. If you are tense and apprehensive, that's what the child will be.*

Q. Why don't ant eaters ever get sick?
A. Because they are full of anti-bodies.

THINGS TO DO BEFORE YOUR CHILD IS ADMITTED TO HOSPITAL

- The child needs to know what will happen to them so they will trust the staff and co-operate. Be open and honest with the child. You have to strike a balance between pretending that the hospital is one big party (because it isn't) and that it is a place to be feared (because it isn't that either).

- Try to be calm. Children can sense when their parents are worried.

- Tell the child the purpose of going into hospital - to get better as soon as possible and go home again. Going into hospital should not be seen by the child as punishment!

- Tell them the truth: that some things may hurt and it's all right to say, "Ouch!" and to cry. Remind them that adults cry too sometimes.

- Let the child ask questions and talk about why s/he is going to or is in hospital. If you don't know the answers, reassure the child that you'll ask the nurses and then get back to them.

- Most hospitals encourage a pre-admission visit, and some have a special program for children. This may include giving them toy stethoscopes and other equipment so the children can become familiar with the doctors' and nurses' 'stuff' and help them to allay their fears.

- Play 'hospitals' at home to familiarise the child with the language, routines and people they may encounter. Buy the child a little bear (dressed in hospital clothes) which you can use to help explain things.

Don't let them put those sticks in your mouth until you know who ate the ice cream!

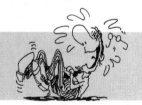

WHAT TO ASK HOSPITAL STAFF

The more informed you are, the more helpful you will be. Here are some questions to ask hospital staff, although you'll probably think of others which relate specifically to your child:

- Are there play facilities and education facilities?
- How many children will be in the unit and what ages are they?
- Will my child be in a cot or a bed?

- Will my child be confined to bed during the day?
- Is there parent accommodation or provision for rooming-in?
- Are meals provided for parents?
- When is the doctor available for information?
- What is the unit's routine (rest periods, meals, etc)?

WHAT TO PACK

Let your child help you to pack. Here are a few suggestions:

- Ask the child to choose one or two favourite toys (including the hospital bear) and a favourite book.
- Photos of family and pets.
- A special outfit to wear home.

NB Label all precious toys and clothes with the child's name.

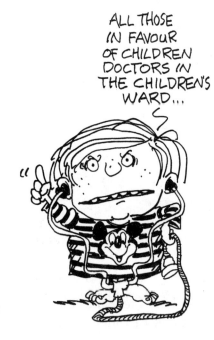

ALL THOSE IN FAVOUR OF CHILDREN DOCTORS IN THE CHILDREN'S WARD...

Arriving at the hospital

Keep in mind that as a parent, you are an essential part of the team. Adopt a confident manner and try to appear in control. Let the nurses know (you may even write these down):

- Your child's name and nickname.
- Foods or drinks your child likes and dislikes (Any allergies to specific foods, drinks and medications).
- Special words the child uses for needing the potty or going to the toilet.
- Whether the child uses a dummy or bottle, or needs to hold a favourite toy or security blanket to eat or get to sleep.

Stay for the doctor to interview you.

Be totally honest with your child; too much information is better than not enough.

Mother

WHEN YOUR CHILD IS HAVING AN OPERATION

There are some excellent books available to help children understand all that's involved in having an operation. Paediatric staff (those who specialise in caring for children) will also be able to discuss your own concerns and provide support and advice. They will also be able to recommend or lend you books or other materials to help both you and the child to prepare for the hospital trip or visit.

Meanwhile, here are a few more hints for nervous mums and dads:

- If possible, arrange for the surgery to be done in the morning, as it is easier to 'fast' a child overnight than to try to keep them away from food or drink during the day.
- Find out if you can accompany your child to the operating theatre and stay there until they are asleep.
- Find out if you can be present in the recovery room when your child is waking.
- Explain the operation and tell the child they will have a 'special sleep'.
- Let the child take a favourite toy to the operating theatre.

Honesty is important. Don't promise what you can't deliver - children have the most incredible memories.

Mother

VISITING CHILDREN IN HOSPITAL

The main worry children have is that their parents will never come back!

- Try to be with your child as much as possible. A visit once a day is important. (Toys and gifts are a poor substitute for your presence.)
- Don't promise that you'll be back and then not return. If you can't come in, phone the unit to let them know, and give them a time that you *know* you can be back at the unit and with the child.
- When you leave the child, tell them that you're leaving - *don't slip away* - then leave quickly and confidently. Put the cot sides up and fasten the catches.

"Nurse, how is that little boy doing, the one who swallowed ten five cent pieces?" Nurse: "No change yet."

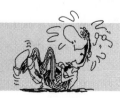

- It's a good idea to let the staff know when you're leaving and when you will return. Expect that your child may cry.
- If siblings visit the child, make sure they don't have a cold or an infection, that they are not too noisy, and that they don't disturb or distress other patients or visitors.
- Leave something of your own for the child to 'look after' until you return.

THINGS TO PLAY WITH
- Homemade puppets help the child to reduce fear by acting out characters.
- Art materials. In particular, painting allows children to express emotions.
- Stuffed dolls and animals are good for 'operating on' by the child.
- Toy medical kits allow for 'acting out' hospital experiences (past, present and planned).
- A personal cassette (or radio cassette) and headphones are great for any age. Take in favourite music, talking books, read-a-longs and even messages you have taped - from you, the child's family, friends, and so on.
- Books, Game Boys, Play Station and Nintendo are all useful distractor.

Have lots of small surprises instead of one large one. For example, pencils In a box can be wrapped individually.

Mother

GOING HOME
- Most children are unsettled for a while when they return home - so expect behavioural changes. They may be clingy and cry if a parent leaves their sight. They may have changes in eating habits, loss of appetite, sleep disturbances, nightmares and perhaps fighting with brothers and sisters. It is important for you to know that your child hasn't been 'spoilt' by the hospital; they just want to be reassured that they are safe and loved.
- Continue your normal routine and discipline for the child.
- Avoid leaving your child for extended periods until they have re-adjusted.
- **Never** use a potential return to hospital or a 'needle' as a threat!
- Encourage the child to work through their emotions by drawing pictures of the hospital experience and by using toys or puppets to explore the characters and situations involved.

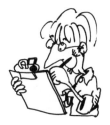

NOTES FOR STAFF

It is often said in paediatrics that, "The kid's not a problem, it's the family!" We agree. Hospitals in general are just not accustomed to involving families, let alone the families who come to us informed and assertive.

Let's face it, the days of 'secret doctor business' and 'secret nurse business' are over. Parents today are more inquisitive and more assertive. They read books, talk to friends and professionals, access the Internet and often know more about their child's condition than you do, especially the chronically ill child or those with a disability.

Those parents who don't do their own research, and who ask you for information, can also be difficult because they are so anxious and disempowered.

We suggest that you *accept parents as an integral part of the healing team* and see them as *colleagues rather than intruders.* This is best demonstrated in your communication, especially when you say the words (with a smile) "Is there anything else I should know about your child?" Listen to their response and hear what they are saying, and say, "Thank you for letting us know."

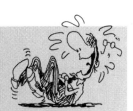

WHAT KIDS WRITE TO GOD:

Dear God, I want to be just like my Daddy when I get big but not with so much hair all over. Sam

Dear God, I bet it is very hard for You to love all of everybody in the whole world. There are only four people in our family and I can never do it. Jessie

Dear God, My brother told me about being born but it doesn't sound right. They're just kidding, aren't they? Marsha

Dear God, Why is Sunday School on Sunday? I thought it was supposed to be our day of rest. Tom L.

Dear God, Instead of letting people die and having to make new ones, why don't You just keep the ones You have now? Jane

Internet

Your Notes

Chapter 20

"You can go home now"

– Leaving hospital

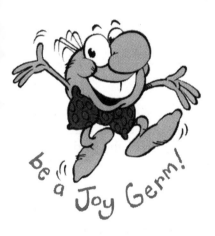

be a Joy Germ!

Preparing to go

Things to check

Leaving against medical advice

Home, sweet home

Day-to-day

Home nursing

Physiotherapy and massage

Getting around inside and outside the house

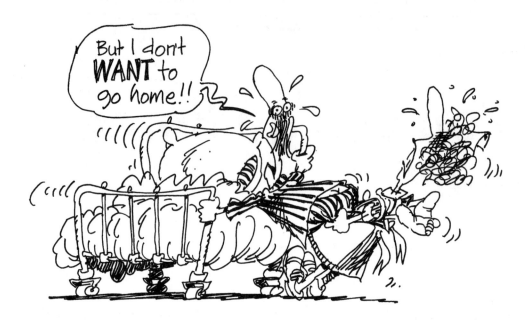

THERE WAS A time when the hardest part of being in hospital was getting out. Now the hardest part is staying in!

It was tough getting a bed in the first place and since then, you've had a funny feeling that there's a game of 'musical beds' in progress and you're not sure of the rules. That's why you've been reluctant to leave your bed to go to the bathroom - in case you come back and find someone else in there with a big smile on their face!

Going home *from* hospital can be more stressful than going *into* hospital. Just the thought of what's waiting for you at home may be enough to make you want to fake a heart attack. You'll have to look after the family, clean up the house, mow the lawn, feed the cats, shop for food, answer the phone, pay bills, answer the door, and get ready to go back to work! All this wouldn't be a problem, but you can't bend over without feeling dizzy, pick things up without that stabbing pain, and you get exhausted just walking to the bathroom.

Short notice

Rarely is going home convenient. The most incovenient time for going home at short notice is 4.00pm, especially on a Friday. It is the most difficult time to organise transport, your medications, and help at home. You should keep in mind that **no-one can make you leave hospital before you feel up to it.**

PREPARING TO GO HOME

It is more than likely that if you are going to need ongoing home care after you leave hospital, a 'discharge plan' (or similar term) will be drawn up by staff in consultation with you and/or your carers. However, if only minimal follow-up care is required, or if staff have been unable to get around to you in time, you may have to do some of this work for yourself. So here goes!

Ask these questions before you leave the hospital and write the answers down:

What:
- you can do to speed your recovery.
- exercises you can do.
- signs to look for that could indicate complications.
- medications to take, when and for how long, and what side effects to look for.
- care you will need at home.
- follow-up tests and procedures are needed and when.

When:
- you can eat normal food.
- you can resume sexual activity.
- you can return to work.
- you need to see your local doctor and/or specialist.

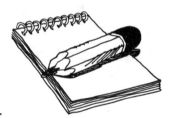

Self-help Groups and Organisations

These groups are worth tracking down and joining. They help people (patients, family and friends) handle the fears and physical challenges caused by medical conditions and surgery. Hospital staff should know what groups exist and how to contact them. If they don't know, contact the hospital social worker, your regional health department, community health centre or your local council.

A hypochondriac is a person who feels bad when he feels good because he's afraid he will feel worse when he feels better.

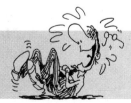

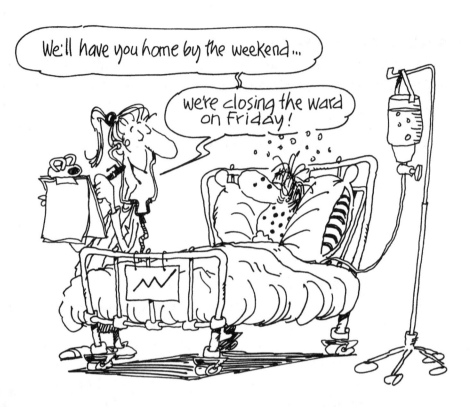

THINGS TO CHECK BEFORE YOU LEAVE THE HOSPITAL

- Medications - your own and those supplied by the hospital.
- Dressings and tapes needed for wound care. (Some hospitals will not supply these, so you will have to make other arrangements ahead of time.)
- Any aides that assist with daily living.
- If needed, reserve a pump for patient-controlled analgesia (PCA) for pain control.
- Any valuables from the hospital safe.
- Letter for your local doctor.
- Sick certificate for work.
- Personal things from your drawers and cupboards.

Make sure you ask questions about new medications or equipment you might need to use once you're home.

District Nurse

Giving feedback to the hospital

If you were satisfied with the service you received, let the staff **know!** Your card or letter may be the one that gives staff a boost on a difficult day. They love it.

On the other hand, they won't love a letter of complaint but make the time to write it so staff know what they need to improve. **Always** finish this letter with something which pleased you about the service you received.

LEAVING HOSPITAL AGAINST MEDICAL ADVICE

You need to know that you have a right to discharge yourself and go home (or to another hospital) if, in spite of the best intentions, things do not work out as you expect in hospital. If your efforts to improve the situation fail, this is your last resort.

As difficult as this seems, it may be better to go than to sit in bed feeling stressed. The hospital staff may ask you to sign a special form which releases them from any responsibility should your condition worsen. *You do not have to sign this form.* If you *do* decide to sign the form, we suggest you write on the form itself the reason you are leaving and that you are not giving up your right to take any legal action that may be necessary.

Leave your account and ask the hospital to mail it to you.

In the meantime, write to the hospital, explaining your reasons for leaving against medical advice. You may also wish to get some legal advice.

HOME, SWEET HOME

Being home can be wonderful - as a relief from the intensely 'medical' atmosphere of the hospital - and relaxing. Or it can be the most stressful part of being ill. In hospital you are the centre of attention. At home, you are more likely to be on your own.

There is a real risk that your family and friends will assume that because you've been sent home, you must be well again. In consequence, you are likely to experience a whole range of emotions which can change from one minute to the next. This is normal!

Here are a few tips for coping when you are at home again.

Go easy on yourself

Most people underestimate the time it takes to get well. Remember - you are recovering from the stress of being in hospital, as well as the stress of your condition. There are some things you will not be able to do and there is no point in getting frustrated and stressed. Surrender to the healing process.

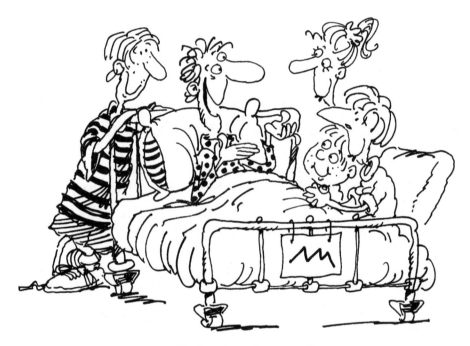

Patient in hospital.

DAY TO DAY

- Get dressed as often as possible to give your brain the message of 'wellness'.
- Make time for laughter.
- Concentrate on the parts of you that are perfect and function well. Look at what you've got left, not what you've lost.
- Think about keeping a diary or journal. It will help you to sort out emotions as you come to terms with your condition, hospitalisation and convalescence.

- At your own pace you can do a heap of things from the 'gunna' file - write those long overdue letters, take up that correspondence course, sort those photographs and put them in the album - all at your own pace and in tune with your body's needs.
- Let your friends and relatives know how they can help you - with light housework, gardening, driving, caring for pets, etc.

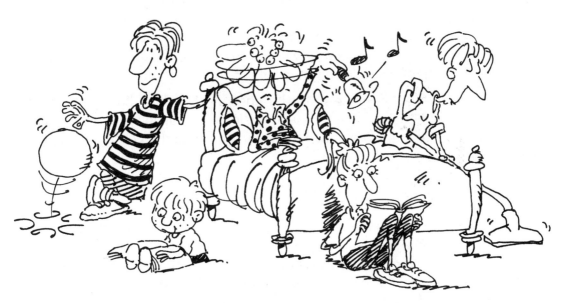

Patient at home.

I can't do all the things I used to do and I've accepted that. If it doesn't get done today, there is always tomorrow, or the next week, or next month. My experience with what I call my 'miracle' has made me realise that people love me for <u>me</u>.

Patient

HOME NURSING

Government-funded nursing, generally known as 'district nursing', is available if you need to continue treatments or you need help with your hygiene needs after leaving hospital. This is a wonderful service, full of committed and caring people. The difficulty they face is trying to meet the increased demand for their services (because of shorter hospital stays) with too few resources.

Your request for their help may be means-tested, and a small fee per visit requested. The hospital (or day surgery centre) should arrange for you to have this support at home. Make sure you mention to the nurses if you do not have anyone at home who can look after you - especially over holidays such as Easter and Christmas. Do this before you leave the hospital so it can be organised, and a 'liaison nurse' who will do this may see you in the hospital. Let them know about other services you already have at home - such as 'Meals-on-Wheels' or 'Home Help' - which can be recommended.

Prepare for the district nurse's visit by ensuring that they have your correct address and telephone number. (Give directions if your house is hard to find.) You should also let them know the best visiting times and if you are going to be out at a time they are due to visit.

The private nurse alternative

Registered Nurses can be hired to look after you during the day and/or at night for any number of hours you require. Another idea is to hire a Registered Nurse as your 'patient advocate' to co-ordinate your treatment and support. This is a good way to reduce the confusion that often occurs when you have several specialists involved in your care, or you're having more tests and treatment.

You can engage any nurse you know or who is recommended to you (provided they are registered), or consult your phone directory under 'Nursing Agencies'.

The people who are expected to look after themselves without support at home include young mothers with children, single people and older people. Many of these people need support just to get through each day.

Community Nurse

Although only 40 and out of hospital after a hysterectomy, I was able to get home help through my local council. It was about three hours a week for six weeks, and cost very few dollars. This meant I didn't have to do awkward and potentially dangerous things like cleaning the bath, or pushing around a heavy vacuum cleaner. And my home help became a friend into the bargain!

Patient

PHYSIOTHERAPY AND MASSAGE

Some people (including doctors) have no idea how helpful physiotherapy and massage can be in getting you well again. Consider visiting a private physiotherapist or masseur, or arrange to have someone come to your home.

Getting vertical was the hardest part. I was feeling 'heady' for weeks, having been on my back for so long.

Patient

GETTING AROUND INSIDE AND OUTSIDE THE HOUSE

Do you need walking aides? Do modifications need to be made to your home, especially the bathroom? Discuss the options available to you with your nursing service, your Case Manager at the hospital, or the home care supervisor at your local council or community health centre.

Make arrangements for someone to drive you to the places you need to go. You could even set up a driving roster amongst your friends and family.

I cooked meals and froze them before I went into hospital. I was glad I did, because I couldn't be bothered cooking after my operation.

Patient

What patients say:

Keep at hand phone numbers for the doctor, ambulance and who you can call if you need help, especially in the middle of the night.

I set up a sub-station (a table) near the bed with things I needed often, such as drinks, snacks, writing paper, phone, books, etc.

I ordered a three week supply of 'Lite n' Easy' meals.   It's a weight reducing food delivery service, but it worked just fine for me.

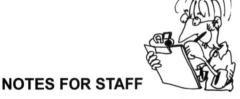

NOTES FOR STAFF

As you know, huge financial incentives exist for getting patients out of hospital as early as possible. Unfortunately, community support services have not been supplemented to deal with this increased workload. Nor have health care professionals in all hospitals developed 'discharge planning' to offset the negative consequences of early discharge. In consequence, the 'revolving door syndrome' exists where patients (especially if they are elderly and/or live alone) go home without proper planning and then have to come back to hospital - often in a poorer condition than when they left.

'Discharge planning' should really start when the patient is admitted, even if you use a checklist with prompt questions about the patient's home situation. District nurses can provide a comprehensive service, provided they have notice that they are needed.

Chapter 21

Enjoy your day
– Be a Joy Germ!

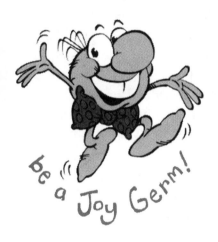

be a Joy Germ!

An outbreak of joy

How to be a Joy Germ

- Be happy

- Be friendly

- Be helpful

- Cheer up hospitals

- Say "Thank you"

- Accept kindness

- Be patient

- Be courteous

joy *n* happiness; delight; great pleasure

joy.ful *adj* expressing or feeling joy; causing happiness; glad

Joy Germ *n* friendly person

DOCTORS ARE NOTORIOUS for running late. They run late for ward rounds, lectures, seeing patients, writing prescriptions and attending meetings! This can cause a lot of stress for the people who are waiting for them, especially the nurses who want to get patients seen and their work finished. Nurses try everything to encourage doctors to do what they want them to do - they ask them, they threaten them, they plot revenge and they bribe them. A typical bribe is a promise not to call a particular doctor at a really inconvenient time - like in the middle of the night!

This is a 'Joy Germ' story about how some nurses at Princess Margaret Hospital in Perth creatively tackled the problem of doctors running late for outpatient clinics. They prepared large sheets of paper on a board showing the names of the doctors, their clinics and their starting times. If the doctor arrived on time, they received a gold star. If they ran ten minutes or more late they had a snail sticker put next to their name. This **attendance competition** was put in the outpatients' foyer for everyone to see and enjoy.

At the time of the competition, we were in the Hospital having lunch with one of the surgeons. At ten minutes to two, he got up from the table, excused himself and said "I'd better go, or I'll be late for outpatients and get a snail!"

This fun way of making doctors more aware of punctuality was well received by the doctors themselves, the nurses and the patients. At the end of three months, prizes were awarded to doctors with the most gold stars and those with the most snails. A bright tie for the winner - and a plate of snails for the doctor who was most often late. This competition improved punctuality by 30 per cent!

AN OUTBREAK OF JOY!

No one would question that the business of hospitals is serious. Yet we know that healing occurs best in a happy environment where people are helpful, flexible and friendly. Our hospitals could be transformed overnight if everyone in them decided to become 'Joy Germs' and act kindly towards each other. Have you noticed how kindness is contagious? When you've received kindness from someone, you just want to pass it on. When this happens we will have an outbreak of joy throughout our hospitals.

Joy has the power to open our hearts, remove fear, instil hope, and foster healing. A truly joyful person transmits energy to all around them. When we collectively start to feel joy, our ability to love each other expands enormously. From this place we can move toward resolving differences between groups of people and hopefully evolve to a level where we feel compassion and care for all life on this planet.

Charlotte Davis

HOW TO BE A JOY GERM

Be friendly, smile and say "Hello"

I say "Hello" to everyone I meet, then I don't have to think whether I will or not.

Teenager

As you walk through a hospital donate a smile to a worthy cause. Make it a habit to smile and say 'Hello' to patients, visitors and staff. This will create a **smile wave** throughout the hospital! When you greet another person and it is not returned, don't take it personally - just remember that some people are worried and distracted and simply don't see you.

We were with Patch Adams one day when he was clowning at Nazareth Nursing Home in Melbourne. He approached a resident, and as he did, the resident's sister who was visiting at the time, said to Patch, "I don't think you'll get much of a response from him." Patch looked at the visitor, smiled and said "Response? I'm not here for the response, I'm here to give." It was a lesson for all of us.

The most revolutionary act anyone can commit is to be publicly happy.

Patch Adams

Decide to be happy

We all have the power to decide how we want to feel each day, so you cannot blame 'the system' for your behaviour in 'the system'.

- Refrain from judging others harshly, whingeing and complaining.
- Look around for kindness and you will find it.
- Look for the good things that people are doing and praise them.
- Be an example of what you want other people to be.
- If you have to work, set a goal to make it a great shift.
- If you're a visitor, be a visiting 'Joy Germ'.
- If you're a patient, know that you have a choice in the way you experience your illness or operation.

The opposite of joy is not suffering, because both can exist together. Its real opposite is despondency and despair.

Joyce Grenfell

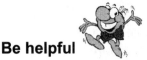

Be helpful

Human beings are designed by nature to depend on each other. Studies suggest that helping other people can reduce stress and boost your immune system! One reason for this is the warmth that comes from people whose gratitude and affection we have inspired. Let the warmth and joy fill you and give you energy to keep doing what you do.

Kindness is the golden chain by which society is bound together.

Goethe

The best exercise for the heart is to bend over backwards for somebody else.

Anon.

   Look for ways you can lend a hand. There are lots of things to do in hospitals that do not require clinical competence. Examples include: holding a door open, carrying something, helping to clean up, assisting a patient with their meal tray and putting fresh water into flower vases. Ask people, "What can I do to help?" You may even decide to become a hospital volunteer.

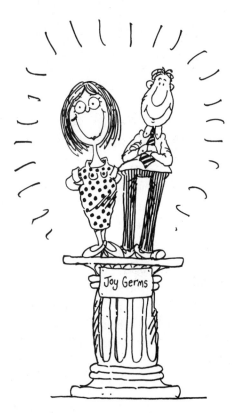

We transformed our staff room from a 'sad room' to a 'glad room' by bringing in things from home we no longer used. We put pictures on the walls, got rid of the rubbish, replaced the cups, put in some magazines and hung some curtains. Next time we're on the night shift we're going to paint it!

Nurses, Dimboola Hospital

Cheer up our hospitals

   The nurses who did this had decided to take the initiative to make improvements and not wait for a 'requisition' and someone else to do it for them.

   There are so many places in our hospitals that could be made a little more cheerful with the help of 'Joy Germ' initiatives.

We remember the nurse who made big *Get Well Soon* signs to put up in her ward, saying, "We don't tell patients what we want them to do!" The same nurse made creative *Fasting* and *Nil By Mouth* signs that had a large crocodile with bandaged jaws!

Another hospital set up a *Happiness Committee* who dressed up in fun clothes and visited patients saying, "We're from the Board of Management and we're here to check if you're happy." The Committee members also arranged for 'Wellness Certificates' to be issued to patients on leaving hospital. In another hospital, an operating theatre nurse hung kites from the ceiling in the corridors for patients to look at as they are wheeled to the theatre.

Perhaps we should look at the colour and creativity of children's hospitals and emulate them in adult hospitals. Would you rather be admitted to 'Starship Hospital' (the name of a children's hospital in Auckland) or 'The Alfred' (the name of an adult hospital in Melbourne)?

Express your gratitude - Say 'Thank you'

There are many ways to thank people in hospital. For example, when you telephone the hospital and it takes a while for people to answer, try saying, "Sounds like you're having a busy day. Thank you for taking my call. May I speak to...?" Whenever we do this, the switchboard staff seem to love it.

- Write notes to various departments in the hospital as they deliver good service to you. For example, pop a note on your meal tray for the kitchen staff, complimenting their food. Thank the cleaning staff for a 'spic and span' room, or for topping up the water in your flower vase. Phone up a local radio station (or the hospital's in-house radio programs) and ask for a 'Thank you' anouncement for staff on your ward, or in the operating theatre, etc.
- Congratulate the hospital shop on their range of goods.
- Give compliments to the people around you.

Laughter is the shock absorber that cushions the blows of life.

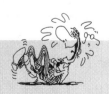

Be creative
- Use chocolate frogs and chocolate fish, *Lifesavers*, a fresh or artificial flower in your correspondence.
- Put gold stars and stickers on requisitions, people and notes (*Slicker Stickers* in Perth have a great range; phone 08-9434 1922).
- Buy (or create your own) 'thank you' cards and use them a lot.

Accept kindness from others
- Be prepared to welcome and receive help from other people.
- If you see someone acting kindly or having some fun - urge them on or get involved yourself. Joy Germs love support.
- Tell people "I've enjoyed our conversation," or "I'm glad we met, you've cheered me up."

Joy is not in things, it is in us.

Anon

Be patient

Impatience causes stress, not only to the person waiting but also the person who may be trying to do their best under difficult circumstances.

Here are some things you can do while you're waiting:
- Start talking to the person next to you.
- Share a joke or funny story.
- Practise smiling: imagine you have an apple on each cheek, then lift your apples.
- Combine this with happy breathing - breathing more fully with every breath you take. Enjoy the surge of endorphins!
- Do some neck exercises: without moving your body, turn your head as far as possible to the right and left. Now do it with your mouth open!
- Think of how you'll compliment the person you're waiting to see.

The best way to cheer yourself is to try to cheer somebody else up.

Mark Twain

Wear something colourful

One way to take the stress out of being in hospital is to wear something a little bit wacky or colourful. It gives people a sign that you are a Joy Germ. Perhaps a coloured scarf, mis-matched socks or earrings, a bright tie, a vivid jumper or a funny hat. We often do this when we visit hospitals and we have found it breaks the ice. The other things we do include giving out 'Have a Happy Day' stickers, *Minties*, or our Joy Germ cards.

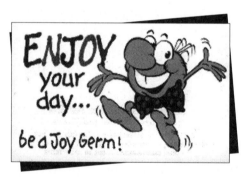

We don't laugh because we are happy. We are happy because we laugh.

William James

Be courteous

- Being courteous is a way of showing that we care about people. It helps people to live and work together smoothly.
- Courtesy is reflected in your attitude, words and actions, which includes saying "Thank you", "Excuse Me", "May I?", "I'm sorry", "May I ask you some questions?" and "Thank you for waiting".
- Introduce yourself, use people's names, look at people when you speak to them, listen attentively, hold a door open, be approachable.

Remember names and use them

People feel important when you use their names. Find out the names of staff members and use them. Especially the person who is looking after you on a particular shift. "May I know your name, nurse?" If you forget, say "Remind me of your name please"

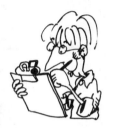

NOTES FOR STAFF

When a doctor sits down for one minute at the bedside to talk, the patient experiences it as five or ten minutes. If the doctor stands in the doorway, the same visit seems like fifteen seconds.

Dr Bernie Siegel

It is not always easy to be a Joy Germ when you are overworked and understaffed, but opportunities do exist. A smile takes a second and saying "Hello" to visitors as you walk through the hospital takes no time at all. Giving praise and a pat on the back to a colleague lets them know that they are doing their best and gives them energy to carry on.

Some of the best hospital units we have seen have been those where visitors and patients are asked for their ideas on how to make improvements. Why not put in a colourful *suggestion box* where you work, or run an *ideas competition,* to solicit ideas from other people? Some of these ideas may not only take the stress out of being in hospital, but they may also save time. **Visit our website: www.chy.com.au** for more ideas on taking the stress out of hospitals.

By Patricia Cameron-Hill & Shayne Yates

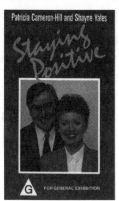

STAYING POSITIVE (video)

This is the most popular video in our range, so if you plan to invest in just one video, this is the one we recommend. It is motivational, uplifting and shows how to take better control of your life and manage tough times. Watch with Chapter 8: Get well soon: the healing power of the mind.

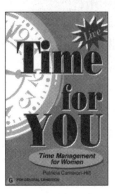

TIME FOR YOU (video)

This video challenges the expectation that women should be able to work full-time and also be responsible for the home. It emphasises the importance of sleep and leisure time for wellness and quality of life. A feature of the video is how to say "No" to unreasonable requests. A great gift for any woman.

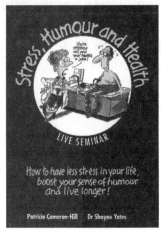

STRESS, HUMOUR AND HEALTH (Four audio cassettes)

We have recorded our most popular seminar on tape so you can have less stress in your life, boost your sense of humour and live longer. This program is a buffet of stress busters seasoned with funny stories and lots of laughs. These tapes complement all chapters of "Doctor, I feel funny" and will go a long way to keeping you well!

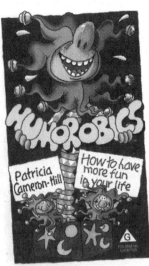

HUMOROBICS (video)

Often described as 'hilarious', this video shows how to boost your sense of humour to reduce stress, recover your health and have more fun in your life. Take with Chapter 14: Laughter medicine! And for Chapter 6: Kiss it better - pain relief.

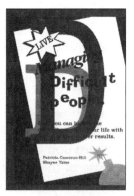

MANAGING DIFFICULT PEOPLE (Four audio cassettes)

This is your chance to share in the fun and laughter of a live seminar as you listen to ideas to boost your self confidence and communication skills. This four audiotape program includes a good helping of assertive techniques to make it easier to ask for what you want. These tapes are a must with Chapter 15: I don't like to make a fuss - speaking up.

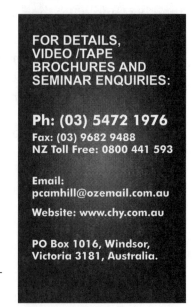

TRAINING VIDEOS

These videos are an easy and effective adjunct to staff education programs in all organisations especially hospitals, wards and units. They are an ideal gift for staff as a way of saying "thank you" or as a way of making needed improvements through education. It has been our experience that where shortfalls in behaviour and/or service exist, they can largely be attributed to lack of staff education.

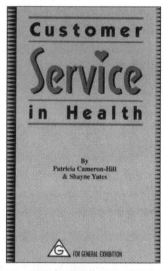

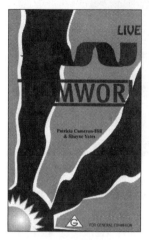

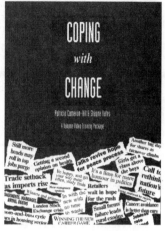

CUSTOMER SERVICE IN HEALTH
(with screening guide)

The key issues of service: attitudes and behaviours are demonstrated in vignettes and role-plays relevant to health care. Facts are combined with fun in three parts: (1) Being happy in the service (2) Understanding people (3) The Seven Service Skills.

TEAMWORK
(with screening guide)

Improving teamwork is one of the biggest concerns in organisations today, and hospitals are no exception. This video shows people how to build a better team by being more considerate and helpful towards each other. Relevant stories and practical ideas are included for each of the easy-to-screen parts:
(1) Attitude (2) Helping others
(3) Giving recognition (4) Fighting fair
(5) Having fun.

COPING WITH CHANGE (with worksheets and screening guide)

Change is a major source of stress for many people. Much of this stress comes from not knowing how to take advantage of the opportunities that come with change. This unique program devotes a 10 minute video to each of the key characteristics of people who thrive in times of change:
(A) Anticipate change (B) Believe in you (C) Continue to learn (D) Decide action. Each video concludes with a summary of options for action.

SEMINARS

Most hospitals would love to have a Cameron-Hill & Yates Seminar but cannot make the funds available to do so. This gives you the chance to show your appreciation of staff in a novel and practical way with a gift of a seminar. These can be presented on a range of topics in a time frame to suit the hospital or department. Topics include: (1) Stress, Humour and Health (2) Customer Service in Health (3) Staying Positive (4) Teamwork (5) Coping with Change (6) Humorobics! The best way of arriving at a suitable topic is to secure the seminar investment, then leave the topic open for negotiation. A free profile video is available to see our presenting style.

Another gift option is to take advantage of our public seminars where staff can attend as individuals or as a group. By contacting Cameron-Hill & Yates Seminars you will know when they are next scheduled in Australia and New Zealand so you can invest in a single or group registration. This is always a welcome and acceptable way of saying "thank you" or celebrating a special occasion.

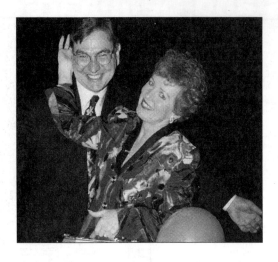

Patricia Cameron-Hill B.App.Sc. (Adv. Nsg.)
Shayne Yates M.B.B.S.

Patricia Cameron-Hill started her career in health care as an Enrolled Nurse at the Repatriation Hospital, Adelaide, and did her General Nurse training at Royal Adelaide Hospital.

After completing a Nursing Degree in 1981, Patricia established a private management consulting business for hospitals and - especially - nursing services. She soon realised that hospital staff themselves were quite capable of making improvements *if* they were given the education and opportunity.

Shayne Yates, after graduating in Medicine from Monash University, spent most of his time working as a doctor in hospitals and private practice. He met Patricia in 1984, and together, they established a seminar business.

Since that time, Patricia and Shayne have presented seminars to a wide range of people including health care professionals, in Australia, New Zealand, Singapore and the United States. Their work has involved visiting hundreds of hospitals and seeing for themselves the challenges they face and how creative staff have dealt with them. Many of these ideas are included in this book and more are recorded on audio tapes and videos produced by Patricia and Shayne especially for health care staff.

Patricia and Shayne now specialise in seminars called 'Stress, Humour and Health' (how to reduce stress, boost your sense of humour and live longer). They present these seminars and have produced tapes and videos for teachers, health care professionals, the corporate sector and the general public.

Patricia and Shayne first heard of the work of the American doctor, Patch Adams, in 1997. Subsequently they invited him to visit New Zealand for the first time and to make a return visit to Australia. His work, wisdom and friendship are a source of inspiration to Patricia and Shayne and encourage them to continue their commitment to making much needed improvements in the health care industry for patients and staff.

Patricia and Shayne are married and now live in Castlemaine, Central Victoria.